I0091384

GET HEALTHY
STAY HEALTHY

A PRACTICAL GUIDE FOR
GOOD HEALTH

DON DURRETT

(Eighth Edition, October 2024)

Copyright © 2018 by Donald David Durrett
All rights reserved.

ISBN: 978-0-692-04093-5

WWW.DONDURRETT.COM

Books by Don Durrett

A Stranger From the Past

Conversations With an Immortal

Finding Your Soul

Finding Your Soul Workbook

Spirit Club

Last of the Gnostics

The Gathering

Ascension Training

Team Creator

Your Soul Explained

The Path Forward

The Demise of America: The coming breakup of the United States, and what will replace it

Kern County: The Path to Secession and a New Constitution

How to Invest in Gold and Silver:
A Complete Guide with a Focus on
Mining Stocks

Post America: A New Constitution

America's Political Cold War: Why
Neither Side Can Win

Your Soul Explained

Are We God?

Good health and good health habits usually go together.

– Don Durrett

CONTENTS

Introduction

I originally published a health book about life extension in 2017. However, I quickly realized that I had limited my audience. The good news was that the material in my life extension book did apply to everyone if I made a few changes. So that is what I have done.

This book is for those who are concerned about their health, but do not want to use rigid methods that are required for life extension. In order to add years and vitality to your life, it requires a lifestyle of optimal health. That type of lifestyle is not easy and not for everyone. This book, however, is for everyone.

I am a layman and not a professional. You can consider any statement that I make in this book as my opinion. The only thing I know about health is from personal experience. I'm writing this book because I feel that my experience and knowledge is worth sharing. The title of this book says that it is a practical guide and that is it what it is, based on my experience.

Take what you want from it and apply it to your life. Hopefully, it will help you to make some changes that improve your health. I believe that good health is a choice and that we are all in charge of our personal health. It comes down to desire and intent. Do you want to be healthy or not? It's usually a choice, and this book helps you to understand what choices are available.

In many ways, this book is a condensed version of a lifetime of learning about health-related issues. I took health seriously in my early twenties and made an effort to understand which foods are healthy. I also began exercising consistently. These two focal points led me to a holistic view of overall health. As you read this book, you will come to see this holistic view. I am constantly learning and expanding my knowledge of what choices I can take to improve or maintain my health.

As you read this book, you will be presented with numerous ideas on how to improve your health and change your health habits. The goal is for you to change your lifestyle so that good health becomes a priority and not just something you take for granted.

The book title begins with Get Healthy. However, that's not really what this book is about. It's more about getting healthier and then maintaining a high level of health. It's intended for people who are already healthy but want to maintain or improve their level of health. If that's your goal, then this book is for you.

I don't think it is hyperbole to state that if you follow the recommendations in this book that not only will you live to be 100, but you will do so in an amazingly healthy way. That's my objective, and it should be yours as well.

Don Durrett 9/27/2018

Chapter One

EAT WELL

Disclaimer: This book includes advice on nutrition. However, I am a layman and have only learned through experience. If you are going to make any changes to your diet, then consultant with your physician.

* * * * *

The most difficult thing to do for good health is to eat well. For some people, it is nearly impossible because of ingrained habits. It is probably the most formidable challenge you will face for improving your health. The irony is that once you change your eating habits, it becomes very easy to follow. The difficulty is in changing them.

Most of you are not going to like this chapter. That's because most of you are likely using food for satiation and not for health. If you want good health, then you will need to learn how to eat to live and to stop living to eat. There's a big difference. Ideally, everything that you consume should sustain good health. Once you achieve this attitude, the battle is won.

I didn't need to do very much research to write this chapter. I have been focusing on healthy eating for decades and I have learned quite a bit. If you take your nutrition seriously, then you will also be able to write this chapter, or something similar. Let's jump in and get started.

Eating well is all about exclusion and inclusion. You need to exclude certain foods and include others. Let's begin with what you need to exclude. Here is the list:

1) Refined sugar and sugar substitutes (except a few listed below).

2) Vegetable and plant-based oils (except a few listed below).

3) Simple carbohydrates (except infrequently).

4) Preservatives and additives (except infrequently).

You need to stop eating sugar on a regular basis, except for fruit and honey. Beet and cane sugar are not as bad as corn sugar, but they should all be avoided as much as possible. Moreover, all artificial sugar substitutes should be avoided. There are a few natural sugar substitutes, such as stevia and chicory, and it's okay to include some foods that include filtered cane sugar when done in low quantities or infrequently.

Why the exclusion of sugar? Because from a nutritional standpoint, it is clearly flawed and should be avoided as much as possible. It's like taking a drug. Sugar raises your blood sugar level, often quite dramatically, and puts stress on the body. The number one reason there is a diabetes epidemic is from the overconsumption of sugar. It's obvious that the body does not like it. In fact, some people consider sugar to be toxic.

A new book just came out called The Case Against Sugar. I haven't read it, but I did read some of the reviews. It's a diatribe against sugar. The story of sugar is steadily turning negative. In my opinion, the consumption of sugar is likely to decrease as more people become aware of its pitfalls.

If you exclude sugar from your diet, you will steadily come to realize that not only do you not need it, but you are glad you stopped eating it. It's kind of like stopping smoking. There is a relief that it is part of your past. This is a surefire sign that it is not good for you. In fact, it will become very difficult to eat pastries and other high sugar content foods. You will get used to saying, "No, thank you," when dessert is offered.

I do occasionally eat foods with sugar, such as at Christmas time. However, this is the rare occasion. I rarely bring sugary foods into my house, except, perhaps, some Italian cookies or banana bread given to me by a family member. On a yearly basis, these are rare events.

Many people are even more strict than me when it comes to sugar consumption. My advice is to be as strict as you can, without going crazy. Recognize sugar's flaws, but also recognize that a little bit won't make a difference to your overall health. It's okay to have dessert once in a while.

Next, exclude vegetable and plant-based oils from your regular diet. The only oils that are healthy are avocado, coconut, and cold-pressed extra-virgin olive oil. Some people even consider olive oil to be unhealthy, but not me, although do not heat up olive oil, and only eat it at room temperature. If you need to cook with heated oil, use avocado oil, coconut oil, or sesame oil.

Note: There are different thoughts on using olive oil or avocado oil for frying. Do your own research. Many researchers think that they are safe for frying. Olive oil has a smoke point at 405 degrees. Sesame oil is at 410 degrees. Coconut oil is a bit lower at 350 degrees. Avocado is best at 520 degrees.

Without vegetable and plant-based oils in your regular diet, this means you can only eat fried foods on rare occasions. You may find that some of the foods you are currently consuming on a regular basis have these oils. I suggest that they be removed from your diet or reduced to an infrequent basis. I still occasionally eat fried food, but only a few times a year.

Both olive oil and avocado oil are mono-unsaturated oils. This makes them healthy to consume at room temperature (in my opinion). Coconut oil is saturated, but has unique properties, making it less susceptible to causing cardiovascular damage, even when heated during cooking. Coconut oil consumed at room temperature is perhaps the healthiest oil. I consider raw coconut to be a superfood, and highly beneficial to the body.

Most vegetable and plant-based oils can create plaque buildup in our arteries, which can lead to heart disease. When vegetable oil is heated, it creates oxidation, which is known to create adverse effects in the body. These are the main culprits for the thousands of heart surgeries that occur in this country. And it's not just fried foods to worry about. Hydrogenated oils, also called trans-fats, are in myriads of processed foods. These can be just as harmful as fried foods.

Whenever you read a food label and see the word oil, you can bet that it is not one of the three good oils that I have listed for regular consumption. More likely, you will see one of the vegetable or plant-based oils listed, or the term, hydrogenated oil. You want to avoid these as much as possible.

The next thing to avoid is simple carbohydrates. These are what many people call comfort foods, such as snacks, chips, pastries, and desserts. Just about every snack or dessert is made from simple carbohydrates – anything that is processed, such as chips, crackers, bread, candy, cereal (nearly all), pastries, pies, cakes, cookies, and soda pop. None of these foods is very nutritious because they are made from processed simple carbs, which generally have low nutrient levels. To make matters worse, they are immediately converted by the process of digestion into blood sugar (glucose) and, often, into fat – if you already have too much sugar in your system. The immediate conversion into blood sugar is why these are the feel-good foods. You can also call them the temptation foods. As I said earlier, sugar is like taking a drug.

Most foods now are labeled with a carbohydrate count. If you read the labels of the foods I listed as simple carbs, you will see that they all have a high carbohydrate count. This is why they can make you fat fairly quickly. Anytime you consume more than approximately 30 grams of carbs at one meal, there is the potential for your blood sugar level to get overloaded. Once you overload, your pancreas will secrete extra insulin to lower the amount of sugar in your blood. The excess sugar goes to the liver, which will create fat from the excess sugar. Basically, your body tells your liver that it has plenty of sugar for energy, and to go ahead and create some fat, in case it needs energy later.

Note: It is difficult to eat a meal with less than 30 grams of carbohydrates. Most of my meals are 50 to 60 grams of carbohydrates. I weigh 160 lbs., so adjust accordingly. I have found this is the right amount of carbohydrates for me. The only reason to stay under 30 grams is if you are trying to lose weight or to ensure that you do not gain weight.

Now you know where nearly all of our fat comes from: the overconsumption of carbohydrates. If you consume less than 30 grams of carbohydrates for a meal, it is nearly impossible for the body to generate excess fat, although you could do it by consuming large quantities of meat or, perhaps, cheese. How people normally gain weight is from overconsuming carbohydrates, and simple carbohydrates are usually the culprits.

So, simple carbs are bad in two ways. First, they have very little nutritious content. Second, once you overload your body with too much sugar, you generate fat.

It's not bad for you to consume simple carbs once in a while. The key is to do it at infrequent times and to not go overboard.

Sure, it won't be nutritious, but you will enjoy it, and I suppose it is an energy source, even though it is comprised of mostly empty calories. A little bit of popcorn at the cinema won't stop your quest for a healthy life, but try to keep it out of your pantry. In fact, it would be a good idea to keep your pantry as bare as possible of simple carbs and processed foods. I have learned that if you keep comfort food in your house, it will get eaten.

The next thing to avoid are preservatives and additives. These are mostly chemicals and not food. When you read a label and don't know what the listed ingredient is, you can bet that it is a preservative or additive. An additive is supposed to make the food either look better or taste better. The worst additive is probably MSG (monosodium glutamate), which the food industry loves, and I detest. It adds flavoring and shelf life, but has several potential negative side effects. It's amazing that this stuff is legal. Google it and find out for yourself.

If MSG is legal, then what other preservatives and additives are we ingesting with our processed foods that are unhealthy? I think we have to assume the worst and avoid them as much as possible. If you are not a label reader, it's time to start.

After you begin reading labels, preservatives and additives will become obvious because they do not sound like natural foods. Sometimes, you will find labels with literally dozens of words that you cannot pronounce. Any food ingredient that you have never heard of, or can't pronounce, is likely to be a preservative or an additive.

Some preservatives to avoid are sulfites, nitrates, BHA, BHT, bromate, and sulfur. These preservatives usually appear as longer words, such as sodium nitrate, sodium sulfite, sodium benzoate, or sulfur dioxide. Anything that has one of these words is suspicious, at best.

Are there any healthy preservatives or additives that the food industry uses? Perhaps, pectin, which is made from fruit, but I'm not aware of any others. And don't trust foods just because they are sold at a health food store, or have an organic label. Many of these foods still contain unhealthy preservatives or additives. Read all labels.

One category not on my exclusion list that many people exclude is some dairy products. There have been studies that indicate that dairy products may cause inflammation, but these studies are not definitive, and people react differently. Milk does have a protein called casein that is very similar to gluten in molecular structure. I have switched from using cow's milk to almond milk because I know that almond milk is healthy, and I'm not sure about cow's milk. I've read that many cows are given pharmaceutical drugs and hormones to keep them from getting sick and to increase their milk production. Plus, I'm not ecstatic about how cows are milked by machines in cramped quarters.

Note: Butter has a negligible amount of casein because butter contains very little protein. Also, butter made from grass-fed cows is actually one of the few healthy saturated fats. I wouldn't cook with butter, but eating it at room temperature is fine.

My suggestion is that if you use dairy in moderation, then it won't curtail your health. I personally would not eat cheese or any other dairy product daily, but I'm not convinced that dairy is bad for everyone. Keep it moderate and infrequent. Pizza a few times a year will not hurt your overall health.

Simple carbs are much worse for you than a little bit of dairy. Where dairy becomes a problem is when you are already consuming a lot of meat, then you tend to get too much cholesterol. Also, many people are lactose intolerant or sensitive to casein. But for the rest of us, we can eat a little bit of butter, cheese, and eggs from time to time (note that eggs are not a dairy product).

At Italian restaurants, I used to pass when the waiter came around to add parmesan cheese to my pasta. Now, I say yes, please. It turns out that hard cheese (aged), such as parmesan and Gouda, is actually good for you. Who knew?

Note: There is no reason to consume cholesterol because the body can create what it needs. Cholesterol is only found in animal products, and those on a vegan diet (which is free of animal products) have been tested for low cholesterol levels. Vegans have been found to have sufficient cholesterol levels.

Another food that is excluded by many is gluten, which generally is associated with wheat products, although it is also found in barley, rye, and malt (unless it is fermented). Gluten is considered to create inflammation. I personally eat wheat on occasion, and consider gluten intolerance to be genetic, and not incurred by everyone. However, it is not a bad idea to limit your gluten exposure.

Because I eat a lot of pasta, I have switched to gluten-free pasta, although I'm probably wasting my time. If pasta was unhealthy for everyone, we would know. I'm half Italian and I've known a lot of Italians who have eaten pasta all of their life. Unless you have a known gluten intolerance, I have my doubts it is unhealthy.

Some gluten-free pasta for you to try: brown rice (Tinkyada), chickpeas (Banza), buckwheat (Soba), and quinoa. These are healthy alternatives to traditional wheat pasta.

Soy and flaxseeds (but not flaxseed oil) contain phytoestrogens. For men (and possibly women), exclude unfermented soy. The reason why is because unfermented soy contains estrogen-like isoflavones. For this reason, consuming too much soy can lower men's testosterone levels. If you are a woman, this shouldn't be a problem, although some research seems to indicate that unfermented soy is unhealthy for either sex. But for a man, phytoestrogens are something better to be avoided in high dosages.

When you dine out, try to avoid fried foods, as well as white and butter sauces. Many of these sauces contain MSG and hydrogenated oils. They will taste great, but your body won't like them. For this reason, try to eat out as little as possible.

* * * * *

Now we get to discuss what to include in your diet. Here is the list:

1) Vegetables.

2) Fruits.

3) Complex carbohydrates.

4) Nuts.

5) Legumes and whole grains.

6) Superfoods.

7) Unsaturated and saturated fats.

8) Meat (optional).

Vegetables are probably the most important food source for a healthy life. The reason why is because they have an abundance of vitamins and minerals that keep you healthy. In fact, vegetables are the best anti-cancer food source (fruits and some teas are a close second). If you are going to consistently obtain nutritional requirements for good health, then vegetables will be required.

You want to eat vegetables every day. I normally eat three vegetables with dinner, with at least one green vegetable. Ideally, you want to eat vegetables raw. However, this is not always possible. For instance, I do not like green beans, broccoli, or asparagus raw and have to steam them. You want to be careful with what you put on vegetables, which I covered previously on which foods to exclude from your diet.

Experiment with different vegetables. Over the years, I have tried many different kinds to find which ones I like the best. Everyone has different taste preferences, and your taste will change over time. You will be surprised how your taste changes once you begin to eat more vegetables and exclude non-nutritious foods.

If you find that you simply do not like vegetables, then you can juice them and combine them with fruit to improve the flavor. This is an ideal way to include them in your diet because juicing can include raw vegetables.

Here is my list of preferred vegetables:

1) Broccoli.

2) Asparagus.

3) Leafy greens (green leaf, romaine, kale, chard, beetroot leaf, spinach, parsley).

4) Green beans.

5) Carrots.

6) Celery.

7) Radishes.

8) Tomatoes.

9) Red and white onions.

10) Brussel sprouts.

11) Zucchini.

12) Artichokes.

13) Cabbage.

14) Green and red bell peppers.

15) Beetroot.

16) Mushrooms.

17) Olives.

18) Cucumber.

19) Shallots.

20) Cauliflower.

* * * * *

The next food source of importance is fruit. Fruits are important because of their antioxidant properties and ability to neutralize free radicals. Fruits are also nutritious and help boost the immune system. I try to eat some type of fruit every day, and most days, I eat two or three different fruits. Do not consume mass quantities of fruit during a single meal because they are high in sugar. A single apple or a single orange is sufficient. A few slices of melon or a couple of handfuls of grapes is plenty for a single serving.

Here is my list of preferred fruits:

1) Apple.

2) Pineapple.

3) Grapefruit.

4) Lemon.

5) Grapes.

6) Melon (cantaloupe, watermelon, honeydew).

7) Dark berries (blueberry, strawberry, blackberry, raspberry).

8) Avocado.

9) Plums.

10) Cherries.

11) Peach.

12) Pear.

13) Orange, tangerine, tangelo.

14) Banana.

15) Apricot.

16) Kiwi.

17) Figs.

18) Mango.

19) Pomegranate.

20) Papaya.

It is okay to replace fresh vegetables or fresh fruit with a frozen source. It turns out that very little nutrition is lost from freezing.

Let's review, so that you have this understood. Every day you need to eat both fruits and vegetables. These are now a daily requirement. You will find that your lifestyle begins to change just from that single decision. You will begin to eat healthily, and you will plan to eat healthily. Plans become habits, and habits become lifestyles.

It's not easy to eat healthily because it requires a lifestyle change. You will find that habits are hard to break. I recommend starting with fruits and vegetables. Once you have your daily habit down of including fruits and vegetables into your diet, the rest of your diet will be easier to change.

* * * * *

The third item to include in your diet is complex carbohydrates. These are good carbohydrates when consumed in moderation. They include pasta, rice, potatoes, and oats. These are the carbohydrates that do not spike your blood sugar the way that simple carbohydrates do. Instead, the body stores these energy sources in an efficient manner, and then disburses them slowly over a period of hours.

This is why marathon runners fill up on these food sources the night before a race.

When you eat complex carbohydrates for dinner, that energy source is available the next day. It is, by far, the most efficient energy source the body uses. The only thing you need to remember about complex carbohydrates is that if you overconsume the number of grams of carbohydrates, then the pancreas releases too much insulin, and the liver can turn the excess carbs into fat. For this reason, it is smart to consume small portions.

I used to eat large portions of pasta or rice. Now I only consume about 30 or 40 grams of complex carbohydrates per meal, which is actually a small portion. This is about the optimal amount to avoid putting stress on the pancreas and avoiding fat creation. It is nearly impossible to generate fat if you keep your carbohydrate intake low.

If you are exercising intensely, you can double your complex carbohydrate consumption and not gain fat. The body is smart enough to "carb load" and not generate fat. The body knows that you plan to use this energy in the near term. Cyclists and long-distance runners consume large quantities of complex carbs and remain thin as a rail.

While potatoes are good carbohydrates, I consider them inferior to rice and pasta. First of all, rice and pasta are easy to cook, which makes it conducive to including them in your daily diet. Second, potatoes are part of the nightshade family (sweet potatoes are not), which are known to cause inflammation in some people. Potatoes can have the same issue as gluten and induce inflammation.

It's okay to eat potatoes, just do it on an infrequent basis. While not all people are affected by inflammation, it's still a possibility. Also, potatoes tend to be cooked in oil or butter. I do like baked potatoes on occasion, and I find that the skin is delicious and nutritious. If you are at a restaurant and want to find something healthy to eat, a good choice is a baked potato and a salad.

I'm probably being too harsh on potatoes. They are an ideal energy source, plus they are high in iodine, which is necessary for a healthy thyroid. In fact, thyroid hormones are important for our energy levels. There are not many food sources that are high in iodine; the other common ones are navy beans and strawberries. If you do not eat a lot of potatoes, then try to consume strawberries on a consistent basis. You can also get iodine from iodized salt, which is salt that has an iodine additive.

For complex carbohydrates, I prefer gluten-free pasta, although I also eat brown rice. My preferred gluten-free kinds of pasta are made out of brown rice, lentils, quinoa, or chickpeas. I do occasionally eat regular wheat pasta when I eat out or at a family dinner.

Some of the longest-living people are from Asia, where white rice is their daily staple. The other thing that they consistently include in their daily diet is a variety of vegetables. While I do not include rice on my superfood list, it is perhaps the best and most efficient source of energy. If there is a perfect food, it's probably rice. If I were Asian, I'm sure I would eat more rice than pasta.

My ideal serving size for rice is one-third cup uncooked, which is 30 grams of complex carbohydrates. For pasta, my ideal serving size is three-quarters cup of uncooked pasta, which contains 35 grams of carbs. It took me a while to adjust to these lower portions. At first, it will feel like you are not eating enough. However, if you are eating complex carbohydrates daily, you will find that is enough to give you energy.

I am five feet, ten inches tall and weigh 160 lbs., so adjust your portions accordingly. I have learned from experience that one-third of a cup of uncooked rice and three-fourths of a cup of uncooked pasta is too much, and I end up feeling too full after eating. Try to learn your ideal portions and consistently use them. Your body is smart enough to remember how to handle your portions.

Note: Measure your complex carbohydrates before cooking to be consistent. Your body is intelligent and will anticipate what it has to digest.

Some nutritionists consider white rice to be empty calories because, other than energy, it does not contain a lot of vitamins. However, it is an excellent source of energy. Brown rice includes bran, which has significant levels of manganese and fiber, making it a more nutritious choice. However, you do not want to eat brown rice every day because it contains small amounts of arsenic and phytic acid (more about this below). I only eat brown rice twice a week. If you want to eat rice more than twice a week, then eat white rice. An important fact about rice is that it can go bad within 30 days if it is exposed to air. For this reason, store your rice in an airtight container.

Occasionally, I will eat one cup of uncooked pasta or more, but these are exceptions when I am eating out (or family meals), and the quality of food is exceptional. These rare splurges are not going to hurt your overall health, but don't make it a habit. Note that after these splurges I always feel like I overate, with a very full stomach. This is another reason to make your own meals as often as possible. You are less likely to overconsume when you cook at home.

Oats are probably the most ignored complex carbohydrate, although some people eat oatmeal for breakfast. If you dislike hot oatmeal, it's easy to make your own cold oat cereal. Combine raw rolled oats, raw chopped almonds, raw sunflower seeds, and raisins (or dried cranberries). Eat it with unsweetened almond milk and blueberries.

Note: Oats need to be soaked in liquid before eating. Do not eat them dry. Soaking them lowers their phytic acid content. Many consider oats to be harmful because they have phytic acid, which can prevent the body from absorbing the vitamins and minerals.

Note: If you eat your cereal with almond milk, I have found that you only need about three ounces of almond milk and the rest water. This gives it the same density as non-fat milk and the flavor is fine. Also, when you mix your almond milk with water it costs half the price.

One of the benefits of eating oats is that it will lower your bad LDL cholesterol levels. There are not many foods that will directly lower your LDL cholesterol. The two most common ones are oats and beans.

You do not need to include complex carbohydrates in your diet every day, but it is a good idea to include them several times a week. Why? Because they will keep you energized, and they are ideal for maintaining your weight. Complex carbohydrates will make you feel full, and you are less likely to snack. I rarely snack and the reason why is because I normally consume complex carbohydrates for breakfast and dinner.

If I have a salad for dinner that excludes complex carbs, I can often tell that I skipped my complex carbs if I exercise the following day. Try to keep your body loaded with complex carbs to keep your energy levels high.

Here is my list of preferred complex carbohydrates:

1) Pasta.
2) Rice.
3) Oats.
4) Russet and red potatoes.
5) Sweet potatoes.

* * * * *

The next category is nuts. I would say fewer people eat raw nuts regularly than exercise regularly. Very few people grasp the nutritional value of nuts. Edgar Cayce, who was called the sleeping prophet, said that eating two or three almonds every day was an excellent way to ensure good health. He even called almonds vitamins.

People think that nuts are fattening. That's a myth. I usually eat nuts daily and I'm thin. People will eat simple carbs, which are fattening, and then skip nuts. As long as you only eat a handful of nuts per serving, you won't gain weight. The key to nut consumption is moderation. The handful rule works extremely well.

I do have one caveat to my handful rule. If you consume your normal amount of calories and then eat an additional handful of nuts for dessert every day, then you will gain weight. In other words, if you overconsume nuts, it is easy to gain weight. However, do not be afraid of gaining weight by consuming nuts as part of your normal diet.

Nuts are very nutritious, and they contain healthy omega-3 and 6 polyunsaturated fatty acids. I find it interesting that nutrition begins with the word nut. Someone is trying to tell us something. Consuming nuts raw is the best way to eat them because they have a higher nutritional content than processed or roasted nuts.

I prefer raw almonds, walnuts, and Brazil nuts, but I eat a lot of different types from time to time. Have you noticed that walnuts are shaped like the brain? Do you think this is a coincidence? Not likely. Mother Nature is trying to tell us something. Also, almonds are actually not a nut. They are seeds. Perhaps this is why they have such a high nutritional value.

Try to eat nuts on a daily basis – one handful a day. A daily basis isn't a requirement, but try to make it a habit of eating raw nuts multiple times per week. Nuts are expensive. For this reason, you have to tell yourself that they are required in your diet. The cheapest form is peanut butter, although peanuts are actually a legume, not a nut. Most other nuts are not cheap. When I go to Trader Joe's, I tend to spend more than I want to on nuts.

Here is my list of preferred nuts/seeds:

1) Raw almonds (seeds).

2) Raw walnuts.

3) Chia seeds (soak first).

4) Pistachios.

5) Raw sunflower seeds.

6) Raw Brazil nuts.

7) Raw macadamia nuts.

8) Raw cacao nuts (seeds).

9) Raw pecans.

10) Hazelnuts.

Are you starting to catch on? You want to consume nutritious food and exclude non-nutritious food. If you exclude nuts from your regular diet, you are depriving yourself of an excellent source of nutrition. As Edgar Cayce said, if you want to be healthy, eat more almonds.

I did not include cashews on my list because of the way so many come to the market. Most cashews are grown in poor countries and workers are subjected to less than favorable working conditions. The reason why is because the shell of a cashew is poisonous on the outside and toxic on the inside! It is dangerous to process and must be done in a careful manner. As you can imagine, workers are not exactly a high priority in some of these countries. There are many ugly stories about what is happening. In India, many cashew workers went on strike to improve working conditions to alleviate the exposure to poisons and toxins. Many people call them blood cashews because of this situation. Until this labor issue is fixed, I have stopped eating them.

In the USA, it can be difficult to find raw, unpasteurized nuts in retail stores. The packaging may say raw, but they probably aren't. Instead, they are likely pasteurized using either steam or fumigation. These processes may kill bacteria, but also reduce the nutritional content.

In California, where nearly all USA almonds and walnuts are produced, all nuts to be sold as raw are pasteurized. In fact, it is illegal for retail stores in California to sell raw, unpasteurized nuts. Yet, most packaging lists the nuts as raw. Currently, as of 2018, a nut label does not have to say if it was pasteurized. In California (and many other states), if you want raw, unpasteurized nuts, then you have to buy them online and they are imported. As you can imagine, raw, imported almonds are expensive.

* * * * *

Next is legumes and whole grains. Legumes are beans. A lot of people do not like beans because they cause gas. However, not eating beans is a mistake. As long as you keep your portions small, you should get very little gas. Moreover, it is usually the foods that you consume with beans that cause gas, such as meat. Try to eat a salad for a meal that contains beans and see if you get any gas.

Note: Raw legumes, grains, and brown rice should all be soaked before cooking. This is required to reduce the phytic acid they contain, which can lead to mineral deficiencies. I won't go into soaking methods, but please do some research if you cook these raw foods.

Pinto beans, black beans, kidney beans, navy beans, and lentils are all highly nutritious. They include significant quantities of fiber, vitamins, minerals, and protein. Also, beans are one of the few foods that lower bad LDL cholesterol. You don't need to eat these on a daily basis, although you can. The key is to include them in your diet on a regular basis.

Here is my list of preferred legumes:

1) Pinto beans.

2) Black beans.

3) Peanuts.

4) Peas.

5) Garbanzo beans (chickpeas).

6) Lentils.

7) Kidney beans.

8) Navy beans.

Peas and peanuts are legumes, but I have a hard time not considering peas to also be a vegetable and peanuts to also be a nut. This is why peas have a high protein content and why peanuts are inexpensive. The best powdered protein, in my opinion, is made from peas. Ironically, they call these vegetable protein powders. I buy vegetable protein powder, and the first ingredient is always peas, which is not a vegetable!

I like unsweetened peanut butter. The Adams and Laura Scudder brands of all-natural unsweetened peanut butter are both unbelievably good. Most people do not recognize the nutritional value of peanut butter. I like to eat it with celery, but it is also good on a sandwich. Peanut butter and jelly with real fruit spread is a healthy combination. Just make sure to go sugar-free and on whole grain bread.

Whole grains are not necessarily a requirement for a regular diet, but they are acceptable. The one thing to be cognizant of is that whole grains are nutritious. In fact, they can be as nutritious as nuts. Often, they include gluten, but not always. Whole grain non-gluten bread or pancakes can be a good addition to your regular diet. My favorite sandwich is almond butter and Smucker's strawberry real fruit spread on Ezekiel sprouted whole grain bread.

I eat Grape-nuts, which is a whole grain cereal. There are many whole grain cereals on the market, and they make an excellent breakfast. I have eaten Grape-nuts for years. Amazingly, it has 45 grams of complex carbohydrate in only a half cup. So, you need to consume small portions. I usually add raisins and sometimes blueberries, which brings it to 55 to 65 grams of carbohydrates.

That's a high carbohydrate count for a daily meal, but it's the first meal of the day and the body is craving food. That's not a bad time to push the limits. I usually can go six to eight hours before I get hungry after this type of breakfast. In fact, I'm rarely hungry after five hours. That shows you how the body likes whole grains and complex carbs.

I get the same response from my body when eating oats for breakfast that I do with whole grains. However, oats have a lower carbohydrate count. There are 29 grams of carbohydrate in a half cup of raw rolled oats. By the way, it's okay to eat raw rolled oats as long as you soak them in a liquid, such as almond milk, before consumption. Most people soak them in hot water to make oatmeal.

* * * * *

Superfoods should be included in your diet because they offer enormous boosts to the immune system and overall health. In actuality, there is no such thing as a superfood. However, over time, more and more people have recognized that certain foods have special nutritional qualities. Thus, they have been deemed to be superfoods. Of course, there is no definitive list of which ones are superfoods, and I'm sure there are scholars who would question some of the foods on my list.

Here is a list of my preferred superfoods:

1) Lemon.

2) Turmeric.

3) Garlic.

4) Ginger.

5) Dark berries (goji, acai, blackberries, pomegranate, blueberries, raspberries).

6) Flax and chia seeds.

7) Green tea, Rooibos tea.

8) Raw cacao nuts.

9) Raw Almonds.

10) Spirulina and chlorella powder.

11) Beetroot.

12) Avocado.

13) Wild Salmon.

14) Coconut.

15) Kelp and seaweed.

16) Hemp hearts.

There are certain foods that are just amazingly nutritious. All of the foods listed above can be included in that category. Turmeric, garlic, and ginger are all very good at reducing inflammation (as is pineapple). Lemon is a magical fruit that helps the body to become pH neutral. It has an alkalizing ability to reduce acidic levels. No other fruit can do this, which I find fascinating. It also is known to detox the body and reduce inflammation.

Dark-colored berries contain polyphenols which have strong antioxidant properties that fight free radicals. They also can reverse cardiovascular disease. One man had nearly total blockage of his heart arteries, and doctors would not operate on him. After several months of eating large quantities of dark berries, his blockages were down to sixty percent. He was now able to have bypass surgery, and the berries saved his life. Just think how good they are at preventing cardiovascular disease.

Flax and chia seeds are like nuts on steroids, as far as nutritional content. Other nuts with high nutritional content are walnuts, Brazil nuts, and pistachios.

Green tea and rooibos tea are high antioxidant drinks.

Cacao nuts are processed into cocoa powder, which is made into chocolate. Raw cacao nuts have a high magnesium content and are very nutritious. They also have high antioxidant properties. The stimulant that gives you a high when you eat chocolate is called theobromine. This is why cacao is called the food of the gods. Some people say that theobromine is the closest thing that replicates the feeling after you have sex. What's amazing is that theobromine is only found in cacao nuts.

Mother Nature did not want people to go crazy eating raw cacao nuts, so she made them toxic to the liver in high dosages. It is recommended that you only eat, at most, five or ten raw cacao nuts a day. To make chocolate, cacao nuts are roasted to remove the toxicity. This also reduces the level of theobromine and nutrition content. However, if you put fifteen or twenty raw cacao nuts in a blender with a frozen banana and eight ounces of water, you will have a tasty chocolate flavored happy drink that lasts for hours. I recommend only drinking this once or twice a week, as it can be addictive and toxic to the liver if over-consumed.

You can also include niacin, lithium orotate, ginseng, and vitamin B-12 to ensure that you have an energetic, happy drink. However, based on my experience, the raw cacao nuts usually do the trick by themselves. You can experiment with some of these ingredients and find out what works for you.

Spirulina and chlorella are perhaps the most densely nutritious foods on the planet. They are both green powders that come from algae. You can literally live off these, which is unbelievable, but true. If you mix these with water, it is enough nutrition to stay alive. How is that for a highly nutritious food source? They are excellent additions for green smoothies. I consider chlorella to be superior to spirulina, but they are very similar.

Beetroot is another nutrition-packed food source. Some people call these beets. They are the hard, reddish-purple vegetables that you see in the produce section of the grocery store, usually chilled. They sometimes have their leaves attached, which is another highly nutritious food source that can be juiced.

The best way to consume most of these superfoods is through juicing or smoothies. Find a way to get as many of these as possible into your regular diet. Note that if you use a blender, you should consume your smoothie immediately. Fruits and vegetables lose nutritional value from blending due to oxidation, and the longer it sits after blending the more nutritional loss accrues. So, you never want to blend and place a smoothie in the refrigerator. Always blend and drink.

Avocados have amazing nutritional qualities. They are loaded with vitamins and are a healthy oil. Plus, they are an excellent way to improve digestion. Eat more guacamole and put them in your salad.

* * * * *

Unsaturated and saturated fats are both required by the body, especially the brain, which is made of mostly fat. You want to consume the majority of your fat through unsaturated oils. These include cold-pressed extra virgin olive oil, avocados, nuts, and seeds. For saturated oil, you can use coconut oil or sesame oil. Other sources include quality butter (grass-fed, if possible), cheese, or egg yolks. As I mentioned earlier, the best way to consume oil is at room temperature and not heated. This also applies to butter, which can be considered an oil.

In case you were not aware, margarine is not butter or even a dairy product. It is made from hydrogenated vegetable oil. For this reason, I would not consider it a substitute for real butter.

If you consume meat, then obtaining saturated fat is not an issue. Animal sources are loaded with saturated fats. Another place to get saturated fat is vegetable oil. This is prevalent in the standard American diet and should be avoided as much as possible.

* * * * *

The last required food source is meat. Of course, this does not apply if you are a vegetarian or vegan. Some people prefer a vegetarian or vegan diet, and others do not. I think this has a lot to do with our blood type and genetics. My blood type is A+, which is very conducive to being a vegetarian. I personally feel healthy as a vegetarian and do not crave meat. If you try to become a vegetarian and you feel awful, then it is probably not something your body is ready for at this time, or if ever.

Note: Type A blood types (35% of the population) find it the easiest to be a vegetarian. Type O blood types (45% of the population) are usually meat eaters. And type B (10% of the population) or other rare blood types, have a better chance of being a vegetarian than Type O. Find out your blood type. If you have type A, then you might want to give vegetarian or vegan a try. Also, if you have a child that doesn't like meat, it might be normal if they have type A blood.

I have known many people who have tried to become a vegetarian, but went back to eating meat. I'll bet many of them had type O blood. Most people who experiment with being a vegetarian end up making some type of dietary change with their meat consumption. Some people end up eating more fish and less red meat, or more chicken and less red meat, but some type of new approach usually results.

If you include meat in your diet, now is the time to reduce its regularity. There is no reason to eat meat on a daily basis, from a nutrition standpoint. The nutritional content of meat is not high enough to be a daily requirement. First of all, meat is not a good energy source, although it is a good source of vitamins, minerals, protein, and iron.

The problem with meat is that it is difficult to digest, especially red meat. By eating meat on a daily basis, you are putting undue stress on your digestive system. Red meat can take days to go through your system, whereas fruit and vegetables can go through in less than 24 hours. Meat acts like a blocker, blocking the path of other foods trying to get through. Do you see how this is not the most optimal way to eat?

There are two other inherent weaknesses with meat. First, it is high in saturated fat. Yes, the body needs saturated fat, but not a lot. Second, it is high in cholesterol. Thus, a high meat-based diet can result in high bad cholesterol (LDL).

If you like meat, then there is no problem consuming it a few times a week, just don't make it a daily habit. The more meat you consume, especially red meat, the more stress you are putting on your digestive system. Sure, the body is an amazing machine and can handle the stress, but you are reducing the likelihood of good health. In fact, you are increasing the likelihood of illness. I was reading recently how a study linked constipation with an array of illnesses. Once you reduce meat from your diet, bowel movements should become much more frequent and consistent.

If you feel that meat is something that you need to have in your diet, then I would suggest fish. The body can digest small amounts of fish much more efficiently than other forms of meat. Plus, fish has omega-3, 6, and 9 fatty acids that are highly nutritious.

The potential for colon cancer has literally exploded in the last few decades. The best way to reduce your risk of colon cancer is to reduce your meat consumption and increase your consumption of vegetables, fruits, nuts, legumes, whole grains, and superfoods. It is my opinion that the best cancer fighter is to live a lifestyle that proactively seeks healthy choices.

There are several replacement foods for meat. Some of these are eaten in pairs to create a complete protein. These pairs include rice and beans, pasta and peas, whole grain bread and peanut butter, hummus and whole wheat pita bread, chlorella/spirulina and nuts or seeds. In addition to these pairs, some foods are complete proteins, such as soy, quinoa, buckwheat, chia seeds, and Ezekiel bread.

Here are some examples of meals that exclude meat and provide a source of protein. The combination of rice and beans is one of my favorite meals and is an excellent way to get protein. One of the reasons for quinoa's popularity is its protein potency. Making protein-rich buckwheat pancakes results in an extremely healthy breakfast. Adding chia seeds or chlorella/spirulina to a smoothie makes an ideal protein drink. A peanut butter sandwich on Ezekiel bread is another potent protein food combination.

* * * * *

Here are a few notes for your diet.

Try to eat less, with smaller portions. Recognize that you are probably eating too much at each meal.

Try to limit your processed food intake. When you go to the grocery store, the vast majority of the food you purchase should not be processed. When you checkout at the grocery store, look at your items and see how many are processed. If it is more than ten percent, then you need to make some changes.

Do not snack. Instead, eat three meals a day and try not to skip meals. You could eat four or five smaller meals if that fits your dietary habits. When you consume smaller meals, it is much easier on your digestive system. I personally prefer three meals a day, plus a dessert of fruit and nuts eaten at least an hour after dinner.

Limit your intake of corn. Most corn (ninety percent or more) sold in the US is now a GMO variety. Also, any processed corn is a starch and a simple carbohydrate.

Limit your intake of chemicals and pesticides. Many people today try to avoid non-organic fruits and vegetables. The main reason why is because most fruits and vegetables are sprayed with pesticides. This is not allowed on organic food. Also, organic food is always non-GMO.

Do not use a microwave oven or use it sparingly. Studies using microwave ovens are concerning from a health standpoint. Did you know that if you put blood in a microwave and then inject it into someone, they will die? Or that if you water a plant using microwaved water, the plant will die? The microscopic pictures of frozen water crystals after being microwaved is also unnerving. Google it. If water looks that ugly, what is happening to the food we microwave?

Do not cook with aluminum pans. There is some evidence that high aluminum levels in the brain correlate to Alzheimer's and dementia. This is another reason not to eat out often.

When eating out, be wary of preservatives, additives, GMOs, and hydrogenated oils.

Try to avoid fast food, if possible, which sometimes can't be avoided. If you are forced to eat fast food, a salad or a baked potato is always a good choice. A veggie bowl with rice at Chipotle is a good choice, or perhaps a veggie sub from Subway. There aren't a lot of good choices out there for fast food. If I'm at an airport, I'll look for Mexican or Chinese food, or perhaps a falafel sandwich.

Chapter Two

DRINK WELL

For some of you, you are going to have to increase your water consumption. Water is the body's cleanser. It cleans out the stomach and intestines. However, it is even more important than that. An amazing fifty to sixty percent of the body is made of water! Cells are actually seventy percent water. We think we are full of blood. No, it's water.

You probably know that the body is constantly rebuilding itself. For instance, cells never last very long. Instead, they are regenerated. Well, all of the water in our body needs to be constantly replaced. For this reason, we should consume mostly water. It should not only be our liquid of choice, but our priority.

How much water are you going to consume on a daily basis, and what is the quality of that water? Well, if you are going to pursue good health, then it better be about 32 ounces of water, and double that would be acceptable. And make sure your water is as pure as possible.

Tap water is nearly always low quality. If it has a bad taste, you can be certain the quality is low. I recommend getting a Zerowater water tester. They are about $20, but very valuable. You can get one on Amazon.com. You can test bottled water, tap water, even restaurant water. Most restaurants, including soda fountains, use filters to avoid a bad taste. For this reason, tap water at most restaurants is usually just as good as bottled water.

Note: In the U.S., fluoride is added to most cities tap water (which is a crime, IMO). You can find out using the Internet if your tap water contains fluoride. Moreover, it is difficult to remove fluoride using filters. Do your own research on how to remove as much as possible.

One thing that surprised me is that not all bottled water is of high quality. In fact, most of them are not. Purchase several brands and test them with your Zerowater tester. You will be surprised at the results, and you might be a bit shocked at the reading for your tap water. Do some research on the internet and you can find out what impurities are in your local water source. It's usually a bit shocking what you discover. You may think that Flint, Michigan, is an outlier, but most municipal water systems have issues.

Fruits and vegetables have water content, but this is not part of your 32-ounce minimum. You need to consume a lot of pure water to flush out your system and keep it detoxified. You need to keep your body detoxed in order to put less stress on it and keep your immune system boosted. Water is the ingredient that keeps everything in working order. Food adds nutrients, but water puts them to work. Water keeps your digestive system clean and detoxed.

When I had my first colonoscopy at age fifty-five, I had zero polyps and my colon was clean as a whistle. One of the reasons why was my daily consumption of water. It is not something that you can skimp on and expect to stay healthy. There are a lot of bad habits that can impact your health, but I would bet that bad water consumption is the most underrated.

If you are not getting 32 ounces of pure water daily, or if that water is contaminated, then you are putting stress on your system. More than that, you are impacting your immune system and limiting your ability to remain healthy.

Note: Some people do not think that 32 ounces of water is enough and recommend doubling that amount. I think 32 ounces is a good minimum for any weight, but drinking twice that amount is not a bad idea.

Believe it or not, water consumption is just as important as the nutrients that you put in your body, or the exercise and rest that you get on a daily basis. You should take your water consumption just as seriously as these other lifestyle choices.

So, for liquid consumption, water should be your primary intake. In fact, on most days, ideally, that should be your primary beverage. Moreover, if you can add fresh-squeezed lemon juice, that is even better. I nearly always include a quarter slice of lemon in my water at dinner. Lemon is a magical fruit that can help you maintain a neutral pH level. It is the only fruit that can accomplish this feat.

I highly recommend that you quit caffeine as a daily regimen if you are under 50. There is no reason to drink stimulants on a daily basis. Some green teas and herbal teas do have significant nutritional benefits, but keep your caffeine intake limited.

Note: In my thirties and forties, I felt no need to consume caffeine. However, once I got into my late fifties, I started to lose some of my youthful vitality. I now consume small quantities of caffeine, such as green tea, matcha, or kombucha, to give myself a boost.

Sodas or anything with sugar or artificial sweeteners are not conducive to good health. Stay away from them.

Fruit drinks need to be treated with caution. First, avoid any with added sugar or artificial sweeteners. Second, keep your consumption to eight ounces or less. These drinks contain high amounts of sugar, even if they are 100% fruit juice. When you drink a glass of orange juice, once you exceed eight ounces, you are eating multiple oranges. Also, unless a fruit drink is freshly squeezed, the nutritional value is reduced.

Note: Dried fruit is a lot like fruit drinks, in that they are very high in sugar content. I would not consider dried fruit as a health food for this reason. I do enjoy raisins and dried apricots, but I tend to limit my dried fruit intake.

Juicing and blending smoothies are ideal ways to increase your nutritional intake and boost your immune system. Both are different, so I will discuss them separately.

Juicing is done with special juicing machines and are not blenders. Juicing machines have the ability to squeeze out enzymes and high nutritional content from fruits and vegetables. I have two different types of juicing machines. One type uses a fast spinning blade that is noisy, and you have to force in the food using a plunger. The other type sucks in the food and is quiet. I recommend the quiet type, which has the added benefit of being easier to clean.

Juice machines can resolve health issues, and are excellent at preventative medicine. If you juice daily, you will boost your immune system significantly. This can heal chronic illnesses that other medications failed to cure. Juicing is so powerful that it can and has cured various cancers. You can watch several documentaries about Dr. Max Gerson and the Gerson Method, which have proven its efficacy. While you likely don't have cancer or a chronic illness, you can still use juicing for boosting your immune system as a preventative measure.

Another juicing documentary to watch is Fat, Sick and Nearly Dead. Joe Cross used juicing to not only heal himself without medication, but he achieved a level of health he never dreamed possible. He has transformed an untold number of lives through his documentary. Even if you get bored halfway through, make sure to watch it to the end. There is quite a surprise in the second half. A four-hundred-pound trucker that Joe meets changes his life. It's quite extraordinary.

I consider juicing to be nutrition on steroids. Some people think that everyone should juice, but I'm not in that group. I do think it is useful for good health, but if you are already healthy, then juicing is probably not necessary to maintain your health. A quality blender to make smoothies is probably sufficient.

I do like to juice a few times a year to give myself a nutritional bump, but juicing on a regular basis seems like overkill when you are already healthy. Again, many people disagree with me and think juicing should be used on a daily or weekly basis to enjoy good health. It's your decision on how much juicing you want to do.

Creating fresh fruit and fresh vegetable smoothies, including many of the superfoods that I listed in the previous chapter, is quite sufficient for boosting your nutrition. Plus, when you drink smoothies, you get all of the fiber that is removed when you use juicing machines. If I had something to do with all of my leftover fiber, I would probably juice more.

I have a friend who has a nutritional smoothie every morning for breakfast. She loads it with superfoods. I highly recommend this for breakfast. Currently, I still prefer whole grain or oat cereal for breakfast because it gives me the energy that I prefer. But smoothies for breakfast make a lot of sense.

There are a lot of nutritional drinks on the market. You have all of the plastic bottle smoothies, which are marketed as health drinks. Some of these are good for you, but many have high sugar content, so read the labels. And depending on if they are pasteurized or made several days ago, most of the nutrition has been lost.

I especially like some of the kombucha brands and flavors. These are fermented drinks made from tea, sugar, bacteria, and yeast. They provide similar benefits that probiotics offer. They are also good at helping your digestion. There is something about the fermentation that the body seems to like.

Jamba Juice and other juice shops that sell health drinks seem to be on the rise. These are ideal because they make their drinks in real time. Habituate these shops as much as possible because it will get you used to drinking healthily. Also, most of these shops allow you to choose what to include. This gives you a chance to add a few superfoods such as chlorella, spirulina, flax seeds, chia seeds, blueberries, and coconut.

I mentioned earlier drinking almond milk with your cereal. All of the "milks" that are made from nuts or coconut are healthy. Coconut/almond is a very good combination, although it usually costs more than the price of almond milk. Hazelnut is very tasty. Hazelnut with chocolate is pretty amazing, although it has sugar added. The vanilla-flavored versions are all tasty. I'm surprised these nut/coconut drinks are not more popular, although, over the past ten years, I have seen an increase in popularity. This trend will continue because they are healthy alternatives to dairy milk.

Coconut water has become popular, and it is highly recommended. Remember, I consider coconut to be a superfood.

Speaking of superfoods, there are many companies that are now selling superfoods in powder form. Vital Reds is a product of concentrated polyphenols. Zuma Juice contains concentrated vegetables, fruits, and superfoods. Both of these products are pricey, but high quality. There seems to be a proliferation of condensed nutrition in powder form.

A few others for you to try are Kachava, AG1 (Athletic Greens)), and Kaged (Outlive 100). I have found that instead of taking one product daily, to take several of them two or three times a week. This multi-product approach is more likely to boost your immune system.

What makes these powders so powerful, other than their high nutritional content, is ease of use. All you need is a packet of powder and some water, and you are instantly revitalized. Call them instant nutrition. This is probably the future of supplements, although this future already exists. I currently mix one of these with water each morning. You can mix them with a fruit juice for even better taste.

If you are drinking a powdered drink or a smoothie, it's very simple to add a tsp. of chlorella or spirulina. Make it a habit.

Chapter Three

TAKE SUPPLEMENTS

This chapter title should be, Take Supplements and Lots of Them. Everyone should be taking a handful of natural, whole food supplements on a daily basis. Why? Because our food quality is atrocious. Our soil has been depleted to the point that we have to eat large quantities to make up for the low nutritional content, and even then, we risk deficiencies. We need to take supplements because it is impossible to eat large enough quantities of food to get the nutrients we need.

One of the reasons people are overweight is that their body is starved for nutrients. This is one reason why people are so hungry and overeat.

While I implore you to take a lot of supplements, I am not suggesting that you exceed a regular dosage of each. Many vitamins can be toxic and dangerous at high dosages. What I am suggesting is taking a wide variety of supplements on a daily basis.

For those of you who are skeptical about the effectiveness of supplements, I have learned that our bodies do, indeed, assimilate vitamins. If I take 100 milligrams of niacin, my body will literally heat up. If I take 500 milligrams, my face will turn red and feel like it's on fire because I am sensitive to niacin. Moreover, many people who find out they are magnesium deficient solve this problem using a supplement.

It is my non-professional opinion that a significant reason why nearly half of all men and one-third of all women in the US will get cancer is because of a poor diet and a lack of supplements. By taking supplements and eating healthily, I believe that the risk of getting cancer is reduced substantially, perhaps even prevented. Moreover, it is a proven fact that many illnesses can be attributed to a mineral or vitamin deficiency.

If you eat healthily to boost your immune system and take supplements to prevent any mineral or vitamin deficiency, you have increased your odds of good health. I've been taking supplements for over forty years, and every year that passes, I realize I should be taking more.

Because of soil depletion, it is nearly impossible to get enough vitamins and minerals from food sources alone. For this reason, you should be including a vitamin and mineral supplement in your daily routine. You can do this with multi-vitamin, or individual vitamin and mineral tablets or capsules. Another option for minerals is liquid mineral supplements, sometimes called colloidal minerals.

Multi-vitamins usually contain iodine, which is a required nutrient for humans. This is the reason we have iodized salt, in which iodine is added. There are a lot of sources for iodine, but vegetarians may skip many of them, such as iodized salt, seafood, kelp, and dairy. There are trace amounts of iodine in vegetables, which comes from the soil. But if the soil is depleted of iodine, then vegetarians can become deficient. This can lead to fatigue, weight gain, and susceptibility to colds. For this reason, an iodine supplement is recommended unless you are getting iodine from what you are eating.

There are trace amounts of iodine in sea salt, but perhaps not enough to prevent a deficiency. If you use sea salt, then you may want to use the iodized version. The extra iodine won't hurt and could help. I have read estimates that up to 40% of the population is deficient in iodine, which is amazing considering how much salt we consume. It's probably not that high, but a lot of people are deficient in this important nutrient.

The vitamins most associated with deficiencies are iodine, magnesium, and vitamin D. You should use a supplement to prevent these deficiencies. The other vitamin that I think is deficient in many people is vitamin C. However, this vitamin can be obtained from consuming fruit on a daily basis.

Note: The body can create its own vitamin D when we are exposed to sunlight. Some believe that we should not take supplements for what the body can create on its own.

The next supplement that is crucial for good health is what are called antioxidants. These reduce free radicals that can induce premature aging. There are myriads of antioxidants, and they occur in most fruits, vegetables, herbs, tea, coffee, and nuts. However, you cannot get enough by eating food alone, because you will have to eat large quantities. You want to consume an ORAC (oxygen radical absorbance capacity) value of 25,000 to 50,000 per day, which is nearly impossible without a supplement.

My current antioxidant supplement has 42,000 ORAC in one pill. There are many different ones on the market.

Here is a partial list of common foods that have high ORAC values that you probably eat quite often:

Garlic, cinnamon, basil, parsley, rosemary, turmeric, ginger, blueberries, blackberries, raspberries, pomegranates, pistachios, almonds, lentils, black beans, pinto beans, artichokes, asparagus, and cranberries. It is a good idea to eat more of them.

Resveratrol is a good antioxidant supplement. It is made from the skin of red and purple grapes. It's also been known to increase energy in rats and mice, and perhaps even have anti-aging properties. Grape seed extract is similar to resveratrol and is also an excellent antioxidant, although not as powerful as resveratrol.

I like to take vitamin C because it is both a strong antioxidant and an immune booster.

I like to take vitamin D and E because we are prone to deficiencies in both because of our poor food sources. If you plan to be outside in the sun, then you can skip your vitamin D supplement on that day. The human body can create its own vitamin D with sun exposure.

I take a cold-pressed flaxseed oil supplement that has omega-3, 6, and 9 fatty acids. I've read that the body can assimilate krill oil much easier than flaxseed oil, and it may be a superior supplement. Also, consider a cod liver oil supplement if you do not eat enough fish or raw nuts. Omega fatty acids are very good for the brain and blood vessels. I used to take fish oil until the Fukushima disaster contaminated a large part of the ocean with plutonium. If you consistently eat a lot of fish, such as salmon, then you probably do not need this supplement.

I am a vegetarian, so I take an iron supplement. An iron deficiency can cause tiredness and impact your blood and immune system. Leafy green vegetables are a good source of iron, but red meat is the best source. Unless you eat red meat, an iron supplement is not a bad idea.

As a vegetarian, I also take a plant-based protein powder supplement in a smoothie. Some vegetarians take these daily, but I only do it twice a week. I find that my regular diet has sufficient protein because I consume a lot of nuts, legumes, and peanut butter, plus my daily breakfast has significant protein. If you consume meat, then it is unlikely that you will get a protein deficiency.

For inflammation: Turmeric, ginger, cinnamon, pineapple, and CBD oil are helpful.

For energy: Resveratrol, vitamin B-12, ginseng, Rhodiola rosea, and polyphenol powders are helpful.

For depression: Niacin, lithium orotate, and lion's mane mushroom are helpful.

For memory: Ginko biloba, huperzine, and rhodiola rosea are helpful. The supplement Alpha Brain works, but it is expensive.

Note: Some of these supplements are made from plants and have been enhanced, which can lead to side effects. Always research the possible side effects of any supplement that you take.

Note: Some people take nootropic supplements for improving memory and cognitive ability (I've used Piracetam, and it works).. However, nootropics have been known to cause significant side effects and are not recommended. Because of their side effects, I consider nootropics to be pharmaceutical drugs, even though they can be purchased over the counter as supplements.

If you have any pain in your body, then you probably also have inflammation. Try this remedy daily and see if the pain goes away: mix one teaspoon of cinnamon with one tablespoon of raw, unfiltered honey. Consume it with an eight-ounce glass of organic pineapple juice, along with two turmeric capsules. Drink lots of pure water. In addition, consider taking C-60 and CBD oil daily (discussed below).

Another anti-inflammation supplement is C-60, also called carbon 60. This is a newly discovered substance without a lot of clinical testing. I know from experience that C-60 helped with inflammation in my shoulder, which went away after about five years of chronic pain. A doctor told me it was inflammation after I had an MRI. He told me to take Aleve (painkiller), which he called an anti-inflammatory. The Aleve didn't work, but the C-60 did. I couldn't do pushups for five years, but now I can do pushups without any pain.

There are several other claimed benefits for C-60, including anti-aging. It's supposedly a very powerful antioxidant. There was a notable rat study that claimed rats lived twice their normal lifespan when taking C-60, but I have not heard of any follow-up studies that confirmed the results. There are risks in consuming C-60 because it is new and has not been thoroughly tested on humans. We don't know if there are any side effects.

The next supplement that potentially helps with inflammation is CBD oil. Many people are using this to combat pain. There are two types of CBD oil, one made from marijuana plants (that contain TCH), and the other from hemp plants (that contain zero TCH).

You can get nearly the same benefits from either plant. However, a highly concentrated CBD oil made from the marijuana plant has potentially additional nutritional properties that the hemp plant does not have. If you live in a state where marijuana is legal, you can grow your own plants and make your own CBD Oil, which is easy to do. All you need is to Google for the instructions.

CBD oil from the hemp plant only has trace amounts (.3% or less) of THC. It's possible to fail a drug test (if they test for trace amounts) if you consume CBD oil made from hemp, but you can't get high. Some people claim that CBD oil from hemp is legal in all 50 states, and others say that it is not. The reason for the controversy is the US government still considers hemp to be illegal to grow and sell, unless there is a specific state law allowing it. Do your own due diligence, depending on in which state you reside.

Perhaps an even more powerful potential benefit of CBD oil is the possible prevention of dementia and Alzheimer's. Early evidence seems to support that CBD oil has a positive impact on the brain as we grow older. There are many other potential benefits of CBD oil, including improved eyesight, and reduced depression and anxiety. Do your own research.

I recently switched from CBD oil to CBDa oil. A company called Nesashemp sells it. The cost is higher, but it is higher quality. CBDa is the main phytocannibanoid compound that offers major health benefits to the body. CBDa has demonstrated superior healing effects compared to CBD. Nesashemp uses high-quality soil and a full cold-preserved hemp extract method. Nesa invented herself, and it is the product of a small business with the goal of producing the highest quality CBDa on the market.

I just realized that I forgot to mention carrots! Have you ever sliced a carrot and noticed that it looks like an eye? That's the Creator's way of telling us to eat carrots for good eye health. Because I strain my eyes from too much computer usage, I eat carrots daily. I like to eat them with hummus (made from chickpeas).

Vitamin A is a good supplement if you don't eat enough carrots. Another supplement that is good for the eyes is lutein. If you have eye strain, then lutein should help. The last supplement for eyes is raw hemp seeds. If you have any eye issues, then research raw hemp seeds.

A good daily (or every other day), supplement for boosting your immune system is the following mixture: 8 cloves of fresh garlic (peel), the same amount of fresh ginger (peel), chop or use a Cuisinart, put in an 8 oz jar, add raw cold-pressed honey and stir. Place in the refrigerator. Eat a 1/2 tsp daily. I like to chew it slowly and put it under my tongue, along with CBD oil.

Another good daily supplement is chaga tea. Chaga is a mushroom that has strong anti-cancer properties. It is also a strong antioxidant. I learned about it from a cancer survivor who drinks two cups of chaga tea a day. You can buy it in a tea bag or powder. I use both, and I am a big fan after reading about it.

I took the following supplements for COVID and did not get vaccinated. I did get COVID, but it felt like a weak cold. I'm glad that I had been taking these supplements.

1) NAC (N-Acetyl-Cysteine) - 600mg 3 days per week. Boosts glutathione, which boosts the immune system against any virus.

Also, eat Brazil nuts and broccoli (food with sulfur). Note: NAC will remove other vitamins/minerals, so only 3 days a week.

2) Vitamin D3 - 5000 units per day. I prefer brands that include K2. Note: Not needed if you are in the sun for 30 minutes.

3) Liposomal Vitamin C - 1500 mg per day. 80% absorption. The best vitamin C you can get.

4) Zinc - 25mg 2 days a week (Chelated for good absorption). This should go with a daily multi-vitamin that also has zinc. Note: Too much zinc can cause issues, so only do extra 2 days week.

5) Selenium - 150mcg 2 days a week. Your daily multi-vitamin should have selenium, so you only need a booster 2 days a week.

6) Quercetin 500mg daily. 3 days a week. Quercetin is known for getting zinc into your cells. Quercetin is not included in multi-vitamins but is included in some of the foods you eat. However, you will not get 500mg from food consumption.

7) Magnesium. 200mg 2 days a week. Your daily multi-vitamin should have magnesium. I supplement that with this extra amount because it is easy to become magnesium deficient. Without enough magnesium, your body cannot absorb vitamin D, so you do not want to be deficient.

Note: There are three different types of magnesium. Try to find a supplement that includes all three.

Other Immune System Supplements

There are a few other plant supplements that people use, and they are quite potent. Here is a short list of the more popular ones.

1. Elderberry.
2. Black seed oil.
3. Cloves.
4. Nettle.
5. Oregano oil.

6. Dandelion root.

7. Echinacea.

8. Astragalus.

9. Golden seal.

* * * * *

The supplements I have listed should only be a starting point. Add whatever else that you think might help with your overall health. I have a few more that I take, but I have not listed them because I am not certain of their benefits. You, too, will likely try several different types, because it's human nature to be curious. There are myriads from which to choose.

* * * * *

Shoulder/Hip/Knee Pain

I came across a YouTube video from a guy who claimed that he rebuilt his knees using diet, supplements, and exercise. I thought I would share it. It's worth a try if you can avoid surgery or get pain relief.

Here are the steps he followed:

Cut out sugar, dairy, alcohol, and processed foods from your diet.

Consider cutting out carbohydrates (this isn't easy for most of us) or limit them.

Consider cutting nightshade vegetables (tomato, peppers, eggplant).

Take collagen, glucosamine, and chondroitin supplements.

Take anti-inflammatory supplements, turmeric, and C-60.

Use intermittent fasting, which helps rebuild cartilage.

Exercise regularly, but without any impact exercises, such as running.

Closing Notes

Dr. Jack Kruse, the neurosurgeon, does not believe we should take supplements for anything the body can generate. He is against taking melatonin and vitamin D as supplements and believes we damage the body's ability to generate both by taking supplements. In the future, I think there will be light generators we can use to generate vitamin D in place of supplements. I have never used melatonin except sometimes when I travel, but I no longer use it as a supplement based on Jack's research.

Chapter Four

EXERCISE

For the majority of people, exercise is not enjoyable and not something that they do on a regular basis. If you fall into this category, then it is time to change your habits and your attitude regarding exercise. You need to perceive it as something that is necessary. Why? Because exercise might be the most important thing that you can do to be healthy and remain healthy.

Not only does exercise promote good health, but it is perhaps the best way to avoid the doctor's office. People will brush their teeth twice a day in order to avoid going to the dentist, but rarely do they exercise to avoid going to the doctor. The best thing you can do to promote health is exercise. Nothing is better as a preventative medicine.

The benefits of exercise are extensive. Here is a partial list:

1) Keeps you strong and vibrant.
2) Helps control your weight and blood sugar levels.
3) Good for your brain (memory, focus, concentration) and mental health.
4) Enhances the quality of sleep.
5) Slows aging.
6) Prevents illness.
7) Prevents injuries.
8) Good for your skin.
9) Gives you energy.
10) Reduces stress (increases dopamine levels).

11. Creates higher rates of respiration which generates melatonin inside the body (this boosts your immune system).

12. Raises your heartbeat and increases blood flow (this boosts your immune system).

Wow, that's an amazing list. You would think nearly everyone would exercise after reading that list. Sadly, only about twenty percent of adults exercise regularly.

The key to success with exercise is making it a part of your lifestyle. It has to be a lifestyle choice, the same as deciding to brush your teeth twice a day. Once the choice has been made, it has to become a part of your weekly routine. Then, when your doctor asks, "How often do you exercise?" you can say, "On a regular basis."

The key to exercising on a regular basis is finding something that you enjoy doing. There are several options. Here is a partial list:

1) Jogging or running.
2) Cycling or an elliptical-type machine.
3) Swimming.
4) Walking or hiking (preferably at a brisk pace or incline).
5) Workouts with weights.
6) Isometric/calisthenic workouts (push-ups, pull-ups, etc.).
7) Aerobic workouts.
8) Sports (that raise your heart rate).
9) Yoga.

If you have not tried everything on this list, then I recommend you try them all to find out which ones you enjoy the most. Think of it this way, you have to pick at least one, so you might as well pick the one you enjoy the most. Without the enjoyment of exercising, you will not have sufficient motivation to make it a lifestyle choice. You can desire good health, but you also have to be motivated. As I like to say, intent is everything, and intent can only come from motivation.

One of my favorite movie scenes is from Man on Fire, in which Denzel Washington helps Dakota Fanning win a swimming race. He asks her, "Trained or untrained?" and she replies, "Trained." He is basically asking her if she is motivated to win.

Your job is to find an exercise, or several, that you prefer. The key is to be consistent (and motivated). Ideally, you want to raise your heart rate for an extended period of at least twenty minutes, twice a week. When you raise your heart rate, you are truly exercising. Doing some form of workout with weights or calisthenics can raise your heart rate, but they usually fail to achieve any aerobic benefits. For this reason, I advise that you find some form of aerobic exercise that you like.

Note: If you are over thirty and have been sedentary, then you may want to consult with your doctor before beginning an aerobic program. If you are over fifty, then you may want to have a treadmill stress test for your heart. I had mine checked at fifty-five, and I had zero blockages.

For those of you who think you can skip the treadmill stress test, I had a friend whose husband died of a heart attack while jogging before he was thirty-five. If you have been sedentary and have recently not done very much aerobic exercise, then a stress test can give you the green light. These tests not only provide the okay to exercise intensely, but they also give you peace of mind that your arteries are clear.

Since my early twenties, I have lifted weights and jogged. This dual-themed exercise program has worked well for me. It achieves both my goal of strength and aerobic exercise. What I have learned from years of experience is that you do not have to do that much for real results. When I was younger, I used to run long distances of six miles or more. I also used to work out in the gym with weights for an hour or longer. I have found out with experience and research that I was wasting my time, and the extra effort did not provide much benefit.

There is very little added benefit once you have raised your heart rate for twenty to thirty minutes, and the same goes for strength workouts. The fact is, less is better. It's much better to increase your intensity and shorten your workouts. Some people have shortened their strength workouts to ten minutes and received enormous benefits. However, I recommend twenty to thirty minutes for both aerobic and strength workouts. You can use this same time frame for swimming, riding a stationary bike, or using an elliptical machine.

Interval workouts have been shown in studies to be the most beneficial. For example, it's much better to exercise at a high intensity, rest, and then repeat. In other words, it is better for your body to swim, jog, or cycle using intervals than to use the same pace throughout your workout. Intervals are more intense, but also much better for you. Repeat after me: intense, rest, intense, rest. That's what interval training is all about.

One optimal method of exercise is raising your heart rate significantly and then using short rest periods, thereby preventing your heart from returning to its normal resting heart rate. Using this method, you can keep your heart rate elevated for an extended period. For example, you can run (or swim or cycle) a lap as fast as you can and then take a short rest. However, do not rest long enough for your heart to return to its normal rate. Then run (swim or cycle) the next lap at a fast pace. Do this to keep your heart rate elevated for twenty minutes.

Another method I like is to begin a weight training workout jogging on a treadmill for ten minutes to raise my heart rate.

Then, after a short rest and without allowing my heart to return to its normal rate, I do a weight exercise at a high intensity. I do another short rest and repeat the weight exercise. During my rest breaks, I monitor my heart by feeling it pounding in my chest to ensure that it remains elevated. Before my heart can return to its normal heart rate, I do the next weight exercise. This may sound ultra-intense, but it really isn't. All you are doing is limiting your rest periods and pushing yourself a bit. I have found that it isn't that much more difficult than a normal weight training workout with very little heart rate elevation.

So, there you go. You only need to exercise for twenty to thirty minutes twice a week to maintain good health. That's all that is required. You can extend workouts to forty minutes or even an hour if you want. Plus, if you add a third or fourth day, that's even better. However, anyone who is exercising five days or more is just having fun. From a health perspective, it's overkill. In fact, too much exercise can lead to chronic injuries, such as knees and shoulders.

Researchers have found that the maximum health effect for the body is running two hours a week. That probably applies to all methods of exercise to some extent. Once you reach a certain level of exercise for a week, the benefits to the body diminish dramatically. Basically, you are wasting your time, unless you are trying to compete in some sport. Yes, you can get faster or stronger with extended exercise, but not healthier.

Give your body a minimum of two workouts a week, although I think four is optimum. Break this down into two strength workouts and two aerobic workouts. Each workout should be somewhere between twenty and forty minutes, although I'm sure some of you will go for an hour. Anything longer than an hour is unnecessary for good health.

One idea for you is to do both your strength and aerobic workouts on the same day. Then you only need to exercise twice a week. If you do both for twenty minutes, you will be done in less than an hour. If you are not an exercise person, then I would recommend this routine. And if you find this to be too much, then you can limit your workouts to twice a week for twenty minutes each. I would consider that to be the minimum for maintaining good health, and it may be insufficient for some people.

Aerobic workouts and strength workouts provide different health benefits. For this reason, it is highly recommended that you do both. For women who do not like strength workouts, I would suggest yoga as an alternative.

You may think that you can avoid both aerobic workouts and strength workouts, and still have a healthy life by being "active." Many people like to perform what I call mild forms of exercise that essentially are neither aerobic nor strength exercises. This would include walking, hiking, and golf. These types of exercise are beneficial, but not sufficient because they do not raise your heart rate. If you are serious about good health, then a combination of aerobic and strength exercises are the most beneficial.

Adding Muscle Mass

Some of you may want to add muscle mass. Added muscle has several benefits, such as increased strength and a higher metabolism, and it is easier to maintain your weight since muscle burns more calories than fat.

For most people, it is difficult to increase muscle mass without protein supplements. People have been trying to gain muscle for decades, so we now know the best way. Ideally, you want to consume 1 gram of protein per pound of body weight. However, you don't want to consume more than 50 grams of protein at one time, and 30 to 40 grams is ideal. If you have a large body, then perhaps 45 grams at a time, and if you have a small body, then perhaps 30 grams at a time.

The best protein supplements contain animal protein because the body is much better at assimilating these supplements. Plant-based proteins are an option, but they don't work as well. The ideal protein supplements are whey proteins. If you consume enough whey protein and work out hard, you should gain a half pound to one pound of muscle in a month.

* * * * *

There are a few things that I have done for the last thirty years that I highly recommend. The first is sit-ups, both forward and reverse. It is my belief that sit-ups are crucial for keeping your back in good working order. I always do sit-ups either before or after my workout. I have occasionally had lower back pain, but my regimen of sit-ups has prevented any chronic pain.

The next thing I have done is to stretch. I usually stretch before I do sit-ups. I believe that stretching prevents injuries. The areas to stretch are your hips, spine, lower back, groin, hamstrings, and calves. If you remain limber, you can stretch all of these areas in about two minutes with relative ease. I personally have never had an injury while stretching, but it is possible to injure yourself if you stretch too hard, so be careful.

You probably haven't thought of stretching your feet, but I recommend stretching your feet tendons using a tennis ball once you turn forty. As you age, the tendons in your feet lose their elasticity. A simple exercise with a tennis ball will stretch your tendons.

What you do is stand on a tennis ball under your bare foot and roll it back and forth. Here's how to do it. While standing, put the ball under your bare left foot. Use your left hand to brace against a table or chair so that you don't fall down. Put as much weight as possible on the ball and roll it from the back of your foot to the front, and then roll it back. Do this twenty or thirty times and then switch feet. If you do this every morning, you will keep your foot tendons stretched and elastic. Plus, you won't have any foot pain.

If you think this foot exercise is a waste of time, have someone who is over fifty years old stand barefooted on a tennis ball. Most people can't because of the intense pain from a lack of elasticity. If you have this pain, it will quickly go away after you begin daily stretching with a tennis ball. What's amazing is that tens of thousands of people have foot pain and don't know about this simple cure.

When you are stretching out your foot tendons, it is an opportune time to do hand-strengthening exercises. I have spent thousands of hours on a computer keyboard in my lifetime, and occasionally, I get pain in my hands and wrists. I have found that by squeezing an inexpensive hand grip, thereby strengthening my hands and wrists, it prevents pain. While I stretch my left foot with the tennis ball, I squeeze a hand grip with my right hand. I squeeze once for each movement of the tennis ball back and forth. Then, when I stand on my right foot, I move the hand grip to my left hand and repeat the exercise. These simultaneous exercises accomplish two things at once, and both exercises are easy to do. Since I began doing this, the occasional pain in my hands and wrists has been significantly reduced and my foot pain is gone.

Note: I started doing the tennis ball exercise after I was diagnosed with plantar fasciitis, which is inflammation of the foot tendon. Plantar fasciitis is common in runners as they age, and I have been a runner for over 30 years. It took more than a year, using the tennis ball stretching technique, for my pain to go away completely. Because plantar fasciitis is difficult to eradicate, it is smart to prevent it from occurring in the first place.

If you do a daily morning exercise with a tennis ball and a hand grip, most of you will prevent any future pain issues with your feet, hands, or wrists. And it will take less than two minutes.

I have one more exercise routine for you to prevent lower back pain. If you have lower back pain, then this exercise should help. I would recommend it as a preventative once you reach forty or fifty, even if you do not have any lower back pain. It takes about three minutes to complete.

1. Stand and spread your feet apart (side to side) as far as possible and still be comfortable.

2. With your knees slightly bent, put your hands on your hips. Lean to your left, while pushing your hip in the opposite direction. This will stretch your groin and hip. Then repeat by leaning to your right and pushing to the left. Do this about 5 to 10 times.

3. In the same position, with your knees slightly bent, lean over until your back is parallel to the ground. Stretch your arms out to each side with your palms facing up. Slowly, move your arms up and down and fly like a bird. This will stretch your shoulders, back, and hamstrings. Do this 10 to 15 times.

4. In the same position, with your knees slightly bent, lean over and touch the ground with your fingers. Lift the heel of one foot while keeping your toes on the ground, which will require you to bend your knee. Then immediately switch to the other leg, thereby raising the heel of the opposite foot. Your toes will always remain on the ground while your heels alternate being lifted. Switch back and forth between legs while your fingers remain touching the ground. This will stretch your hamstrings and back. Do this 20 to 30 times.

5. Still leaning over, with your feet wide apart and knees slightly bent, grab your ankles and pull, stretching your back. Lean down to get a good stretch. Do this 2 or 3 times.

6. Still leaning over, with your feet wide apart and knees slightly bent, take your right hand and grab your left foot, and pull. This will stretch your back. Repeat by taking your left hand and grabbing your right foot, and pull. Do this 2 or 3 times.

7. Stand with your feet close together, lean over with your knees slightly bent, and grab your ankles. Rock back and forth on your feet, raising your heels and then your toes as high as you can. This will stretch your hamstrings, calves, and back. Do this 5 to 10 times.

8. Do the same exercise as in number 7, only this time, bend your knees enough to place your fingers on the floor. Do this 5 to 10 times.

9. With your feet about shoulder width apart and pointing outward, squat to the floor as far as you can. This will be difficult for the first few weeks until you get used to it. This is called the Asian squat. It will stretch out your back and keep your hips limber. Try to do it for at least one minute a day. I try to push my legs apart using my elbows, while rocking side to side, putting stress on my hips.

10. Do pushups until failure. I have found that this strengthens not only my arms, but also my core (which helps your back). If you are over 50, this is highly recommended. Note: I prefer to do pushups using Perfect Pushup handles and gloves, which reduces strain on your wrists, and makes the pushups easier to do (more range of motion).

I've done the tennis ball, hand grip, and stretching for more than a year now and I doubt that I will ever stop. It only takes five minutes, first thing in the morning, and the benefits are substantial.

Chapter Five

REST

This chapter could have been titled Sleep because sleep is where we get most of our rest. However, sleep is only part of the answer. Most people do not consciously think about getting enough rest. You can get enough sleep and still not get enough rest. If you work all the time, then you are probably not getting enough rest.

Work can wear us out. We work for a paycheck, but we also work around the house. Women often work harder than men because they have more hats to wear. My mom was a working mother, and she did all of the shopping and cooked all of the meals. She worked twice as hard as my dad. It's still the same for many working women.

Many people work a significant amount of time without sufficient rest. These long hours of working eventually add up and impact our health. In fact, most people are not aware that this burden of working long hours is impacting their health. If people who are working all hours of the day could find a way to relax and rest, they could be much healthier.

If this is you, then perhaps, add more exercise to your life. Your exercise routines can give you a chance to relax. Other ways include spending more time socializing or spending time with family and friends. Find some outlets that take you away from work. Too much work is going to wear you out and impact your health.

If you don't have an overwhelming work burden, then your only rest nemesis is getting enough sleep. Some people can live on six hours of sleep, some people even less. Most of us need at least seven hours of sleep, and some of us need eight, or more.

This is something that you have to learn on your own. Everyone should know what their ideal sleep requirement is and then try to consistently hit that number. Moreover, to keep your body rested, you do not want to confuse it by living on a variable sleep schedule. If you are consistent, then your body will be consistently rested. This is one important key to good health.

Now, everything I have said about rest is common sense. However, just like exercise, it is a lifestyle choice. You choose to be rested. It's a decision that you personally make. Many people have the philosophy of "I only live once, and I'll sleep when I die." Well, those are not the people who will remain healthy.

Stick to your sleep schedule and stay rested. Your health will benefit.

The key to rest is to stay rested and to have a routine that keeps you rested. If you get run down and tired, then take the time to recharge and do not continue in that state. Better yet, do not allow yourself to get run down. Know your limits and adhere to them. Stay rested.

Here are the top five reasons for a reduced lifespan:

1) Cigarettes.
2) Drug and alcohol abuse.
3) Obesity.
4) Illness.
5) Lack of sleep.

The first four items are obvious, but what is a lack of sleep doing on that list? Until recently, there had been very little research done regarding sleep. Now we know that the body is actually very active during sleep, especially the brain. The process of rejuvenation during sleep is quite complex. It turns out that the brain does just as much work when we are asleep as when we are awake. Moreover, a deficient amount of sleep can be detrimental to both our health and longevity.

It's amazing that people will eat a healthy diet and then deprive themselves of sleep. Or, consistently exercise and then forget to sleep.

Find out how much sleep you need so that you are not drowsy during the day, and then consistently sleep that many hours. Normally that is at least seven hours, with some people needing a bit less or a bit more. I personally need at least eight and wish I could get by on less. I can get by on less than eight, but I can tell that I am not completely refreshed during the day, or I will feel sleepy before bedtime. A refreshed body will tell you your optimal number of hours of sleep.

One thing to be aware of about sleep is that not all sleep is equal. There is something called rapid eye movement (REM) sleep, which is different than deep sleep. The body cycles in and out of REM sleep throughout the night and you only REM sleep twelve to fifteen minutes per hour. The more hours of sleep you get, the more cycles of REM sleep you receive. The average person gets about ninety minutes of REM sleep each night.

Because REM sleep is the most revitalizing, you want to eliminate anything that can prevent it. The first things to eliminate are excessive light and sound. Find out if you are sensitive to light by making your bedroom completely pitch black for two weeks and see if it helps. I did this test and found no difference. I actually prefer to sleep with some light in the room.

You can also try using earplugs and a sleep mask and see if they help. Next, make sure the room temperature is between 68 and 78 degrees. Do not consume caffeine, chocolate, alcohol, sugar, or heavy foods within four hours of bedtime. Lastly, consider the air quality in the room.

Many of us are highly concerned about the quality of our water and then neglect the quality of the air in our homes. Air quality can impact both our sleep and our health. The first thing to check is the humidity level. You can buy a humidity tester for $10 on Amazon.com. You want your level to be around fifty percent for sleeping. For those of you who live in areas of high humidity, you can control your bedroom humidity by purchasing a dehumidifier. And for those of you in dry climates, you can add a humidifier if your bedroom humidity is significantly below fifty percent.

If you live in humid climates, then mold is always a concern, and you should have your house periodically checked by a professional. It's never a bad idea to add an air purifier to a bedroom, although they are never noise-free. One solution is to run them during the day and turn them off at night.

Another idea to consider is removing the carpeting from your bedroom. Most carpets tend to decrease air quality. Another is to make sure that your mattress and pillows are both non-toxic. Shop for non-toxic items the same way you shop for non-GMO products. Look for labels that say non-toxic.

Another mattress issue can be heat. Some mattresses warm up by our body temperature. I remember staying at hotel and waking up in the middle of the night from being too hot. The mattress had become warm and did not reflect the air temperature. If that happens to you, get a new mattress.

If you have trouble sleeping, the first thing to eliminate is any stimulants from your diet, such as caffeine. You will feel tired at first and, perhaps, tired quite often. However, that tiredness will lead to more restful sleep and a more revitalized body. I often fall asleep within five minutes of when my head hits the pillow. A big reason is the lack of stimulants.

If you get run down from a lack of sleep, sleeping extra hours will help, but don't make this a habit. Constantly sleeping extra hours is probably a sign that you are not getting enough rest. For good health, you want to strive for a consistently rested body. The key, of course, is getting enough sleep on a nightly basis.

The next thing to help with sleeping is exercise. If you exercise vigorously, it will tire you out and help with sleep. I have found that exercise and sleep go hand in hand. They both help each other.

Another thing that is useful is reading. If you have trouble sleeping, turn off the TV or computer and read. Tire out your mind. If you find yourself reading a lot to fall asleep, then consider buying a bedroom light that has reduced blue spectrum (or no blue light). These are now easy to find. Just Google sleep lights.

Since I mentioned lights, it's probably a good idea for me to mention that LED lighting can impact sleep. LED lighting is primarily a blue light with an intensity that is about five times that found in nature. These intense blue lights are actually stimulating and can keep you from easily falling asleep. Exposing yourself to bright LED lights before bedtime is counter-productive to falling asleep. Conversely, they are great for waking up in the morning. The best light sources before bed are incandescent and halogen lights or reduced blue spectrum LEDs.

A new bed is always a good idea to try for better sleep.

Sounds can help. Millions of people download various sounds that help induce sleep. In fact, there is a new product called Dreem that provides sounds that have been proven to induce sleep.

There was a strange sleep device is called Sense, but the company went out of business. They sold a smart device that would monitor your room for anything that could impact your sleep. It would even answer questions about the environment of the room and if something needed to be changed. I'm sure another company will soon come out with something similar.

Two other products you can try are Nucalm and Headspace.

As you would expect, there are websites that want to help you with your sleep problem. Just Google sleep programs.

If you have tried all of the above and still have trouble sleeping, then you can try to use a supplement. There are three supplements that are useful for inducing sleep: tryptophan, valerian root extract, and melatonin. All of these can be purchased as vitamin supplements. Since they are inexpensive, try all three and find out which one works best for you. Also, do a Google search and research each one.

Note: It is never a good practice to become dependent on a supplement for your nightly sleep. They should only be used on random occasions, such as when you are traveling. For good health, you want to consistently be able to get a good night's sleep without the need for a sleep supplement. As mentioned previously, Dr. Jack Kruse thinks it is unhealthy to use melatonin supplements. .

Chapter Six

REDUCE STRESS

There is a saying that stress is a killer. I agree with that. For this reason, you have to find ways to reduce stress. The ideal way is through a good marriage, which has been proven to increase your lifespan. If you don't have a good marriage, the next best way to reduce stress is through positive social interaction. If you are consistently laughing with your friends and family, then the odds are good that your stress levels are low.

If you don't have one of those factors in your life, then get a pet, preferably a dog or a cat. A good pet can reduce your stress levels almost as well as a fellow human. My cat and I communicate frequently. From my perspective, we have a relationship that requires constant engagement. She might as well be a human because she has more emotion than some people I know. When I talk to her, she looks at me and I know that she understands. Often, when I won't let her be on my lap, she bites my feet. If that's not an expression of anger, I don't know what is. And you should see her eyes light up when I ask her if she wants to play hide and seek. Have you ever watched a cat run and hide? It's the funniest thing you ever saw, and it reduces stress like you would not believe.

So, social interaction with humans or animals is probably the best thing to reduce stress. However, there are other things that you can do. Exercise is very good for reducing stress, and that is already on your agenda. Walking and hiking outside, or in nature, are also useful. Going to the movies or a concert helps. Attending conferences is a nice outlet, as are vacations. Hobbies are useful.

Religion or spirituality helps. Reading is another stress remover. What do all of these things have in common? They are all relaxing.

The key to reducing stress is preventing it from reaching extreme levels. Stress causes cortisol to release from the adrenal glands. In chronic cases of stress, people release high levels of cortisol on a daily basis. This is really bad for your health. Ideally, you want to limit the amount of cortisol that you release. Less is better.

You never know when stress is going to arise or how you will respond. I would think that everyone has felt its effects at some point in their life. My first experience was when I was in fifth grade, and I was afraid of a bully who was a couple of years older than me. I thought he was going to kill me. It was awful. In hindsight, he never laid a hand on me, and the stress was self-created.

It turns out that nearly all stress is self-created. The exceptions are traumas that are usually not our fault, such as an accident. Stress is always fear run amok. It's a fear that won't leave you alone. It's a mindset that is the opposite of how you want to be. For good health, you want to live with levity, joy, and peace of mind. That's the low-stress state that you want to strive to achieve.

Depression is a form of stress and should be treated. Often depression is repressed anger, and unless we can find joy and purpose in our lives, depression is always lurking. While we can generally know what is impacting our health, we are often blind to the effects of our thoughts.

As I mentioned previously, stress is usually self-created. So, if it is self-created, then it should be preventable. One way to achieve a low-stress state of mind is to let go of willfulness. Instead of directing your life in a perpetual state of willfulness, live with trust and go with the flow. This is somewhat counterintuitive to how we are taught to live. However, instead of trying to direct your life, accept what comes your way. Instead of living with will, live with humility and gratitude. Most people are consumed with stress because they are always trying to direct their lives or are afraid of potential outcomes that are out of their control. They refuse to let go and surrender. They always have a plan and then attempt to control the plan's outcome in a continual act of will.

Less will correlates to less stress. One easy way to reduce your will is to replace the word me with the word we. When you think in terms of we, stress has a way of diminishing. It's when we focus on ourselves that stress seems to appear.

How many people get stressed out because every detail in their life isn't going perfectly? This is from willfulness. Do you see how willfulness is stressful? Do you see how trying to control your life is stressful? Let go and surrender. Live in the now and go with the flow. Don't dwell on the past or worry about the future. Trust that it will work out. That's how you reduce stress. The more you can live in the now, the better off you will be from a good health standpoint.

When I was about twenty years of age, I took a trip to Mexico with some friends. One of my friends had a beach house that his parents owned. While we were down there, I was amazed by these children who lived in a nearby house that had a dirt floor and no electricity. I had no idea that people in Mexico lived in such extreme poverty. What stunned me was their smiling faces. They were enjoying life more than we were. Now, how was that possible? We were on vacation, having the time of our lives. It was us that were supposed to be experiencing happiness, not them.

I thought about that experience for years before I figured it out. Those children were happy because they only cared about the present moment. They didn't care about their past or their future. They didn't care about what they didn't have, only about what was important, which was a loving family. They lived with humility and gratitude for what they had. They were living one day at a time and enjoying the outcome, whatever it was.

I still remember the smile on that ten-year-old boy's face. I was not as happy as he was, not even close. Why? Because I was trying to control my life. I was trying to create my own happiness. At that time, I had no idea that the secret to happiness is to let go and surrender. Once you stop forcing your will onto the future, you will be amazed at how stress becomes less of a factor in your life.

We need to become like that little boy who had nothing, but still felt like the happiest person on the planet. When you reach that same realization, stress will have a hard time finding you.

One method of obtaining this type of mindset is eliminating stuff that you do not need. Try to simplify your life. There are various strategies to obtain simplification. One is to toss out anything that you no longer use. Clean out your garage and storage areas with the intent of tossing out all non-essential items. Every few years, review your wardrobe and eliminate anything that you no longer intend to wear. Make it a proactive part of your life to continuously simplify your life.

Why simplification? Who do you think has more stress, someone with myriads of stuff that they do not use, or someone who only keeps what he uses? Which one do you think has a better handle on their life? Can we measure someone's stress level by the cleanliness of their garage? Probably.

Another method to use is meditation. The secret to meditation is keeping your mind quiet, or silent. This is not easy to learn how to do, but it can be very effective at reducing stress. Perhaps the best time to meditate is when you wake up in the morning. If you quiet your mind for five or ten minutes, that can set the tone for the rest of the day. Consider reading a book that shows you how to meditate. I would recommended *Right Concentration* by Leigh Brasington.

So, use the various methods that I have given you to reduce stress, but more than that, find a way to keep stress out of your life. Stop worrying about the future and trying to control your life. Instead, trust that everything will work out for the best. Live with humility and gratitude. Count your blessings every day and put a smile on your face. If you can do that, then you will be amazed at how you can control your stress.

Life only gives us two things: lessons and opportunities. All of the drama we create is from not recognizing that we are having either a lesson or an opportunity. If you feel stressed, try to figure out what lesson you are learning. Then recognize that you won't get a lesson that you can't handle.

Have you ever noticed that when you are doing something that you enjoy, such as socializing with friends and family, that your mind is present? Or, if you are doing one of the activities that I listed earlier, that your mind is present? When you are engaged in an activity, your mind is always present. This is why these activities are stress reducers. It's only when you start projecting into the future or dwelling on the past, that stress comes into being.

Now that you know what triggers stress, you can try to keep your mind from running you ragged.

Let's end this chapter with a bit of levity. Two of the most joyful things that we do are stress reducers. They are laughter and sex. Studies show that people who laugh more and have more sex, live longer. If they live longer, then laughing and sex are probably good for your health. Makes sense to me. Hugh Hefner is ninety and still going strong. Coincidence? Probably not. Lol.

Chapter Seven

NO DRUGS OR CHEMICALS

Humans love their drugs. Alcohol is a huge business, as is nicotine and caffeine. All three are billion-dollar industries. Marijuana is also becoming very popular, with state after state legalizing it. Caffeine might be the most abused drug of all. I wonder how many people use caffeine to feel good in the morning and alcohol to feel good at night?

Ideally, you want to exclude drugs from your body if your goal is good health. Although, it's okay to consume drugs in moderation and still maintain good health. The key is not to make it a daily habit. You need to treat drugs similarly to the way you approach nutrition. It's okay to have a piece of cake once in a while, but it's not something you want to do on a daily basis.

If you eat well and exercise regularly, and then consistently consume drugs, that is counterproductive to your goal of good health. Drugs shock the system and put stress on the natural state of well-being. The body is resilient enough to handle a daily cup of coffee or a nightly glass of wine with very little residual impact. However, over time, the stress impinging on the body adds up and impacts our health.

There is a common misconception that a daily cup of coffee or a nightly glass of wine is good for you. It is true that both contain polyphenols, which are good for you. However, asking your body to adapt to your drug of choice is not good for overall health. Ideally, your body wants to maintain a state of well-being. And trust me when I say that, when you speed up (caffeine) or slow down (alcohol) your system, that is not a state of well-being.

Medications are also drugs, but they require a doctor's prescription (except for over-the-counter drugs). These also put stress on your system. Today, our ingestion of medications has become an epidemic. A generation ago, we did not consume mass quantities of medications. Today, it's something like one in two Americans are on some form of medication. It's so bad that, if you are over fifty, then you are probably on at least one prescription. This epidemic is clearly related to what we consume.

I'm not going to list all of the medications that people are taking today. I'm going to make this simple. Medications put the same stress on the body that legal and illegal drugs do. For this reason, ideally, you do not want to consume them on a regular basis. Try whatever you can do to be medication free. Do this with your doctor's help if you are using a prescription medication. I know that some people are dependent on anti-depressants and other psychiatric medications. Be very careful removing those from your daily routine without your doctor's help.

The goal of good health is to maintain a state of well-being. In my opinion, anything that we ingest that is not natural is probably impacting our well-being. The key is to find a way to get healthy without the need for anything non-natural.

Chapter Eight

Good Habits

I've already mentioned several good habits in the previous chapters. I'll repeat some of them here.

1) Eat well.
2) Drink well.
3) Take supplements.
4) Exercise.
5) Rest.
6) Reduce your stress.
7) Don't take drugs.
8) Breathe properly.
9. Get sunlight.
10. Take care of your teeth.

For eating and drinking, get in the habit of limiting your caloric intake per meal. This is not easy to do, but is required to maintain your weight. Make it a habit to avoid snacking or eating processed foods. Make it a habit to drink 32 ounces of pure water daily. Make it a habit to eat fruits and vegetables daily.

Those are just a few habits for eating and drinking, but there are dozens of others. Over time, try to adopt good eating and drinking habits.

There are two habits for supplements that I would recommend. The first is to take them daily. The second is to constantly experiment and find out what works for you.

Make it a habit to exercise weekly and stretch daily (especially if you're over fifty).

Make it a habit to get enough sleep.

Make it a habit to monitor your stress levels and proactively keep them down.

Make it a habit to avoid drugs.

I have found that, as you add good habits, they seem to become part of your lifestyle. What ends up happening, over time, is that you come to realize that you are living a lifestyle that focuses on good health. I don't think you start out that way, but, eventually, that is what it becomes.

The good news is that each good habit tends to support adding more good habits. It's difficult to have a good health habit and not have it lead to additional good habits. They tend to feed on each other.

A good starting point is to begin exercising twice a week. Once that habit is firmly established, begin to eat better. Use these two foundations to steadily improve your health and your focus on utilizing good health habits. It will take at least a year to learn how to eat better and form new eating habits. Be patient and take it slow. Try to slowly eliminate certain foods from your diet. Over time, you will begin to see a change.

After about a year, if you have established new habits of exercising regularly and eating better, you can begin to add supplements. In year two, you can firmly establish your new lifestyle of good health. This is where you improve your habits and become more committed to good health.

By year three, you should be practicing all seven good habits listed at the beginning of this chapter. I don't think anyone who is currently not living a healthy lifestyle can obtain one in a single year. In fact, for most of you, it will take three to five years to firmly establish a lifestyle of good health.

The reason for the long duration is our programming. We have been programmed to believe that we don't have to proactively focus on our health. Most of us grew up eating fast food and processed food. Eliminating those won't happen overnight. For most of us, exercise was considered optional for good health. Now it is a requirement. Thinking about rest and stress in terms of our overall health is not something many of us thought about while growing up. Now we have to think about aspects of our lives that we used to take for granted from a health standpoint.

Changing our behavior and the way we view health are big changes to our lifestyle. This is why you have to take it slow. Don't try to live a healthy lifestyle overnight, because the odds of succeeding are very low. You have to do it in steps, with one minor change after another.

Exercise is probably the easiest habit to adopt because it can be scheduled. You can plan to do a workout two or three times a week relatively easily. All you then need to do is be consistent and not quit.

Your diet will take much more effort to change and must be done over a longer period of time. If you are overweight, then attempt to reach your ideal weight and maintain it there.

Here are some tips on losing weight:

The supplements that can help you lose weight are acai berries (usually in a capsule or powder), chia seeds, hemp seeds, and apple cider vinegar. Try all of these for a month each and see which one works best for you. Also, before you take them, read about the side effects and effectiveness of each.

I have found that I lose weight naturally if I eat my normal meals but reduce my nut consumption. I literally begin to get skinny without trying. If I reduce my nightly dessert of eating a handful of raw walnuts, I begin to lose weight. A handful is only about 300 calories per day. Thus, with just a small reduction in calories, you can lose weight.

I think the best diet is to eat a healthy diet with a somewhat restricted calorie intake. Eat three meals a day, but reduce your calories by 300 to 500. Then, once you reach your ideal weight, add back the missing calories.

Note: If you have difficulty losing weight, Dr. Jack Kruse has a paleolithic diet that might be worth trying. It's very simple to follow, and you don't have to starve yourself or restrict caloric intake. His patients have had success using it. He personally lost 150 pounds in a few months using it. Here are the steps:

1) Eat three meals a day and do not snack. At each meal, restrict your carbohydrate intake to less than 25 grams. Consume 50 to 75 grams of protein, including high fat intake (he recommends a lot of coconut oil).

2) Eat breakfast shortly after you wake up and have dinner 4-5 hours before going to sleep.

3) Exercise regularly.

My diet is very simple, and I eat mostly the same thing every week. For breakfast, I currently eat whole-grain cereal, oatmeal, or granola with a mixture of almond milk and water. I usually add raisins and blueberries for flavor and added nutrition. For lunch, I currently eat either a handful of raw almonds, a Kachava blended replacement meal, or an almond butter and real fruit spread sandwich on sprouted grain Ezekiel bread, with an apple. For dinner, I rotate three different meals, all of which consist of vegetables and complex carbohydrates. They are all very simple meals, usually consumed with pure water.

I know what you are thinking. I can't eat like that! Perhaps not, but you can simplify your diet and begin to exclude processed foods and excess meat consumption. The best way to lose weight is to eat your normal diet but with fewer calories consumed each day. As I said earlier, intent is everything.

* * * * *

Supplements will come naturally as you improve your diet and want to get better nutrition and prevent vitamin and mineral deficiencies.

Rest and stress reduction will come last and become more important as you adhere to a holistic healthy lifestyle.

There are a few additional habits that I do and have not yet mentioned.

The first is keeping my teeth clean. Most of you are probably good at this, but not all of you. I think it is imperative to brush twice a day and floss at least once a day. I also strongly recommend using an Oral-B electronic toothbrush since it works so well. I rinse with one of the mouthwash brands to reduce bacteria after I floss. If you rinse with mouthwash, it is recommended to rinse with water afterward. A dental hygienist told me to rinse with water if I use mouthwash because it's not good to keep the mouthwash on your teeth.

Another thing you can do for your teeth is rinse with one teaspoon of coconut oil. This is called oil pulling. However, you need to do this for 10 to 15 minutes to be effective. I do this when I take a shower in the morning. Coconut oil will kill any bacteria in your mouth and remove plaque. Plus, your teeth will feel clean, and you will need fewer cleanings at the dentist. It also has an amazing side effect of adding oil to your skin. I used to get dry hands and dry feet, but not anymore. The frequency is up to you. Some people do this daily, and others do it weekly. I try to do it every other day to keep my hands from getting dry.

Note: Do not spit the coconut oil down the drain because it is an oil. Most water is recycled, and you do not need to make their job more difficult.

The second habit is keeping your ears clean and free of wax. You can purchase inexpensive ear-cleaning fluid at any drugstore. It only takes about ten minutes and works great. This can be done once a month or once a quarter. When you go to the doctor, ask him or her to check your ears for wax. If you clean them yourself, then they should be clear of wax.

The third is keeping your colon clean. You can purchase colon cleanse products (powder or capsules) that will clean your colon. I like to do this every few months as a colon cancer preventative. If you eat meat, then you could do it more frequently.

The fourth is to breathe properly. For most of us, breathing is not something we think about. Instead, we let our body breathe on its own. However, it turns out that many of us are not breathing correctly. Many people are over-breathing and taking around 10 bps (breaths per second), when the ideal breath is 5.5 bps. This has been thoroughly scientifically researched. A good book on this topic is Breath by James Nestor. It's a good read and is guaranteed to surprise you. Anyone who is asthmatic (8% of the population) or has any breathing issues, needs to read this book. Although, I highly recommend it to everyone.

What researchers have found is that breathing less is better for your health. Fewer breaths mean fewer heartbeats per minute and lower blood pressure. Amazingly, it also likely means a longer life. Indeed, proper breathing can extend your life and keep you healthy.

The ideal breath is an inhale for 5.5 seconds and then an exhale of 5.5 seconds. This results in 5.5 bps. This perfect breath has been used by yogis and monks for thousands of years after it was discovered to improve your health.

Why does this ideal breath work better than 8 bps or 10 bps? Ironically, the more you breathe in oxygen, the less the lungs absorb. And even worse, the body exhibits stress when it thinks it is getting too much oxygen. This stress causes the heart to pump more blood than is necessary and your blood pressure to rise. Also, the body is highly intricate and any stress on the body reverberates to other systems, such as how it handles stress and anxiety. As you can imagine, there is an impact throughout the body. Thus, over-breathing is bad!

What is amazing is that the yogis and monks figured this out long before scientists proved it. Not only is over-breathing bad for you, but too much mouth breathing is even worse. It's okay to occasionally mouth breathe, but keep it to a minimum and try to always breathe through your nose. Nestor's book does an excellent job of explaining why slow nose breathing is so important to our health.

So, breathe less and always breathe through your nose. This will reduce stress on the body and extend your life.

The fifth habit is to get enough sunshine. Dr. Jack Kruse, who I have mentioned previously, says that UV light and red light from the sun are crucial for good health. Get outside as much as possible. He especially recommends getting up and watching the sunrise. I don't know what is special about this, but if you are an early riser, it is recommended. This light is very potent, according to Kruse.

On final tidbit from Kruse. He says that blue light lowers our dopamine and can make us lethargic and unmotivated. Nearly all of the manmade light we use today is blue light, including our light bulbs, TVs, computers, laptops, and phones. Ouch.

Perhaps the last health habit to learn is stubbornness and persistence. This is the habit where you focus on your health, and nothing is going to stop you. Once you achieve this habit, you have won. Anything that is going to impact your health will be shunned and excluded to a high degree. You may stay out late for an occasional party, but this will be the exception. In fact, nearly anything that impacts your health negatively will become a rare event. Once you become stubborn with your health, it will become the focal point of your life, and anything that impacts your health will not be ignored.

The bad news for a healthy lifestyle is that many of your family and friends won't understand your focus and commitment to good health. For this reason, you will occasionally get ostracized and perhaps get labeled as selfish or strange. What they don't realize is that people who practice good health are helping those around them and society. Good health is a win-win. It's a win for those who practice it, and it's a win for society as health issues are reduced.

I want to share the results of a Harvard University study that was performed on 123,000 volunteers for longevity. They found that if people followed five habits (see list below), they would live an extra ten years. Being proactively healthy is not the norm, but it is rewarding. Note that number three on this list is the hardest and most important habit. If you want to remain healthy and live a long life, then you have to exercise regularly (unless you have excellent genes).

1) Follow a healthy diet.

2) Control your weight.

3) Exercise Regularly.

4) Drink in moderation.

5) Do not smoke.

In addition to physical health, you need to think about your mental health and reduced stress levels. It is a known fact that we can make ourselves sick with our thoughts. Have you ever thought about what you need for happiness?

Some people can be happy simply from the joy of being alive; however, for most of us, we need a bit more. The average person requires three things to be happy:

1) Good Health (this book helps with this requirement).

2) Sustenance (financial stability).

3) Some form of social interaction.

Each of these has different levels of satisfaction. For the first, you can have perfect health or an ailment that you can deal with. For the second, we can be satisfied with having less, but there is a point where not having enough financial stability is stressful. For the third, some of us are okay with very little social interaction, while many of us need a lot.

The key to happiness is recognizing when all three of these are satiated. This should engender gratitude that you are being fulfilled. Every morning, you should recognize that lucky me, I have all three!

Now, here is the most important part of mental health: there is no number four! To be happy, you don't need anything else besides the three requirements I listed. If you think you need to achieve something to be happy, such as owning a big house or having more money, you are deluding yourself. That's not what will make you happy. This is why many affluent people are miserable, depressed, or stressed out. How many successful rock stars or celebrities ended up with drug or alcohol problems? Achievement clearly didn't make them happy.

So, if you want to feel happy (all the time), recognize that you already have the three things required for happiness.

Some will disagree and say that in order to be happy one must achieve something in this lifetime, and that the people who are the most content have succeeded at life, and that they have earned their happiness. I say, baloney. To repeat, you don't achieve happiness. Instead, you recognize it as the gift of life with heartfelt gratitude.

Everyone has a life purpose, which we have to figure out, but our life purpose doesn't need to create our happiness. In fact, our life purpose is usually challenging. We need to learn to be happy in spite of our challenges and lessons. When we can do that, our health will benefit immensely.

Of course, there are varying degrees of happiness, but baseline happiness, where negative or depressive thoughts do not impact your health, is fairly easy to attain. As long as you don't have a serious health issue or you are not financially destitute, you should be able to maintain a degree of constantly positive thoughts.

It's also possible to dramatically improve your mental health by making changes to how you think about life. For instance, instead of thinking that life creates challenges (where you are a victim), you can see challenges as opportunities. I like to think that life only offers us blessings and opportunities and that we should embrace both. This is not easy to do and takes some work. It's similar to changing your diet. You have to begin to embrace challenges as opportunities and recognize them as something you are creating for a reason. Instead of seeing yourself as a victim, you need to see yourself as someone who is learning a lesson, which is beneficial.

Another piece of the happiness/mental health puzzle is what gives you contentment. This will be different for everyone and has a degree of achievement built into it. So, while you may have to achieve higher levels of contentment, that is only the cherry on top and should not prevent you from experiencing happiness.

To be happy, you have to embrace the magic of life. Instead of seeing life from a poor-me perspective, you have to see it as something that is being given to you and that you are in constant receptivity. Life is one constant gift that keeps giving until you take your last breath. So, ultimately, happiness is the recognition of gratitude that your life was given to you, and it is the lack of gratitude that causes all of our mental health issues.

Mental health and physical health are the most important aspects of our lives, yet we are forced to learn them on our own. Neither are taught in school as required subjects. Most people are poorly educated in both subjects. This is why most people are not in optimum physical or mental health. The irony is that they could be with just a little bit of education and motivation.

I recommend that you go back and re-read this section on mental health and embrace it. The mind is perhaps the most important factor that keeps us healthy. Without strong mental health, the odds are low that you will attempt to keep yourself in optimum health.

Chapter Nine

CANCER PREVENTION
/ LIFE EXTENSION

The previous chapters are focused on cancer prevention and life extension, but I wanted to narrow that focus in this final chapter. There are specific foods, supplements, and methods that I use specifically for cancer prevention and life extension. I have not had cancer and feel youthful, so I think they are working.

This is the chapter where you decide to make a lifestyle decision. Some people eat to live, and others live to eat. There is a big difference between the two. You have to decide whether to take care of your body or not. You can try to do it partially, but in the end, that's probably not going to work effectively.

Most people live to have fun, and food is part of that fun. Their mentality is that you only live once, so let's enjoy it. If that is your mindset, then you are taking a risk with your health. Unless you make a decision to take care of your body, the odds of getting cancer increase dramatically. Conversely, if you follow this chapter closely, those odds are reduced dramatically.

Dr. Brooke Goldner is a specialist in autoimmune disease. She is the author of three best-selling books, Goodbye Lupus, Goodbye Autoimmune Disease, and Green Smoothie Recipes to Kick-Start Your Health and Healing. Her website is www.goodbyelupus.com.

What's fascinating about Dr. Goldner is her story. She came down with Lupus as a teenager and had a serious case of it for about ten years. It was so bad that she almost died. Then, when she was going to get married, she asked her fiancé if he would give her a diet to lose weight to fit into her wedding dress.

She followed his diet for about 6 weeks and lost the weight to fit into her dress. Then after she got married, she suddenly felt great. She went to her doctor to have tests to find out why she felt so good: her Lupus was gone! Not only that, but it never returned.

I'm writing this because the diet she followed can be used intermittently to boost anyone's immune system. That's basically how she healed herself. Ironically, it was similar to the diet that Dr. Max Gerson (the Gerson Method) used to treat cancer patients. That treatment is illegal in the US because nutrition is not considered a proper way to treat cancer. It is used today in foreign countries, such as Mexico and Japan.

What is the magical diet? Dr Gerson used juicing. Dr. Goldner uses smoothies. What they have in common is a high intake of liquefied green vegetables. It turns out that the body's immune system can be boosted using food alone. This is a fabulous way to prevent cancer and keep your health at an optimum level.

Radiation Balancing

Use this method to remove radiation from your body and to injest baking soda, which is known to prevent cancer.

How often? I do it monthly, but you can do it weekly if you prefer.

32 oz water (distilled).

1 tsp sea salt.

1 tsp baking soda.

Mix thoroughly.

Drink about 8 to 16 oz's every 4 hours.

Cancer Prevention Foods

1) Beverages: chaga mushroom tea, green tea, black tea, jasmine tea, licorice tea, peppermint tea, ginseng tea, matcha tea, rooibos tea, 100% pomegranate juice, 100% cranberry juice, Ryze mushroom tea, Mud Water (cacao powder and mushrooms), pure water.

   Frequency: Daily

   Note: I rotate my morning beverages. Currently, I have three that I rotate for better nutrition.

   Note: I like to use a mixture of teas. For instance, I like chaga, licorice, and green tea all at once. Another good combination is chaga, rooibos, and ginger. Ryze.com has an excellent matcha-mushroom tea that is fabulous.

   Note: Bottled water is actually unhealthy. Why? Microplastics leach into the water. So, try to use a filter at home instead.

   Note: Use honey, coconut, or fruit as a sweetener.

2) Vegetables: broccoli, onion, spinach, kale, green beans, asparagus, tomato, carrot, dark green lettuce, peas, cabbage, celery.

   Frequency: At least one daily, and most once a week

   Note: I like to eat my broccoli in a thick soup. Boil it in water, then put it in a blender after removing most of the water. Add some salt and serve.

3) Nuts/seeds/legumes: Brazil nuts, almonds, walnuts, peanuts, macadamia nuts, pistachio nuts, hummus, peanut butter (without sugar), black beans, pumpkin seeds, sunflower seeds, pecans.

Frequency: Daily (except black beans weekly)

Note: One serving of nuts should fit in your closed hand.

Note: I prefer carrots with hummus and celery with peanut butter as an appetizer before dinner.

Note: I prefer a handful of nuts before bed. I rotate the variety of nuts for better nutrition.

4) Garlic/Ginger/Honey

   Mix the following together:

   1/6 fresh chopped garlic

   1/6 fresh chopped ginger

   2/3 cold-pressed honey

   Frequency: Daily or two or three times a week (1 tsp)

   Note: This will remain fresh in your refrigerator for at least two weeks.

5) Celtic Sea Salt, Himalayan Pink Salt, black pepper, cyan pepper.

   Note: I put this on my vegetables and red pasta sauce.

   Note: Purchase your salt and pepper in kernels or chunks and use a mill to grind them right before eating

   Note: For salt, pepper, herbs, or supplements, always buy organic.

6) Fruit: strawberry, blueberry, blackberry, raspberry, kiwi, banana, apple, mango, grapefruit, lemon, orange, watermelon, peach, plum, nectarine, apricot, cherries.

Frequency: Daily

Note: If you are lazy like me, a quarter slice of grapefruit is always an easy choice before bed.

Note: Keep your portions small because fruit does contain sugar.

7) Oatmeal: add cinnamon, raisins, blueberries, chia seeds, hemp hearts, bee pollen, goji berries, flax seeds, dried cranberries.

Frequency: Daily for breakfast

Note: I generally only add about five toppings to my oatmeal, but gave you several options.

8) Miscellaneous: Here is a list of important foods that need to be mentioned. EVOO (extra virgin olive oil), cocoa powder or dark chocolate (without sugar), brown rice, lion's mane mushrooms, shitake mushrooms, basil, peppermint, gouda cheese, whole grains, fish oil, yogurt (without sugar), honey, and avocado.

Frequency: Weekly

9) Guacamole: 2 small avocados, 1 small Roma tomato (sliced), 1/8 inch slice of white onion (chopped), garlic salt. Mix in a bowl and serve with tortilla chips.

Frequency: Weekly

10) Cyan pepper: 1 tsp EVOO (extra virgin olive oil), ¼ tsp cyan pepper, ¼ slice lemon (squeezed). Mix in a small glass. Drink.

Frequency: 2-3 times a week (in the morning)

Cancer Prevention / Life Extension Supplements

1) Essential vitamins (A, B, C, D3+K2, magnesium, zinc, minerals)

   Magnesium in the morning (Malate or Citrate)

   Magnesium before bed (Orotate or Glycinate)

   Note: You can now get vitamin D3+K2 in liquid form, which I have been using.

2) Condensed nutritional powders (reds and greens)

   Note: I consider Kachava a nutritional powder, although it is considered a meal replacement.

   Note: You can add 1 tsp of apple cider vinegar to your powder drinks.

3) Turmeric

4) Taurine

5) CBD Oil

6) Colloidal Minerals

7) Resveratrol

8) Quercetin

9) Selenium

10) NAC (N-acetyl cysteine)

Cancer Prevention / Life Extension Methods

1) Avoid sugar (honey, maple syrup, and fruit are okay)

2) Avoid processed foods

3) Avoid alcohol/smoking/drugs

4) Avoid overeating

   Note: You should not feel full after a meal.

5) Exercise (at least twice a week)

Note: 1-2 hours a week of aerobic exercise. 1-2 days a week of strength training.

Note: After age 50, do stretching, pushups, and pullups daily.

6) Rest (lots of sleep)

7) Take supplements (boost your immune system)

Frequency: Daily

8) Read (exercise your brain)

Frequency: Daily

9) Juicing

Note: This is optional, but a good habit.

10) Donate blood.

This generates new blood cells and revitalizes your body.

Note: This is optional, but a good habit. It requires a 48-hour recovery period.

Cancer Treatment

As I stated at the beginning of this book, I am not a doctor and learned everything you have read as a layperson. However, if come down with cancer, I would try all of these known treatment methods.

1. Intravenous Vitamin C.

2. Vitamin D.

3. Zinc.

4. Mebendazole.

5. Fenbendazole.

6. Low sugar, low carbohydrate diet.

7. Green juicing / green smoothies.

8. Ivermectin.

9. Baking soda, sea salt, and water.

10. Dandelion root.

11. Oxygenated water.

12. Essiac herbal tea.

13. Match - Mushroom tea.

14. CBD/CBDa oil.

As mentioned before, I am not a doctor. This is information that I have come across. It is up to you to do your own due diligence.

BOOK REVIEW REQUEST

If you enjoyed this book and think that others would benefit, please write a review on Amazon. Most readers rely on reviews to make their decision. It's sort of a catch-22 for me as a writer. I need reviews to sell books, but I need to sell books to get reviews.

www.ingramcontent.com/pod-product-compliance
Lightning Source LLC
Chambersburg PA
CBHW072151020426
42334CB00018B/1959